PREFACE

This book is an aid for the trainee preparing for examinations. We have included several styles of question, including the multiple choice question, to reflect the range of examination techniques used world-wide.

We hope this book will bring a little light relief to the drudgery of reading thick tomes that all students must suffer. All the authors have attempted to keep the subject matter in the sphere of the everyday life of an ENT surgeon. In-depth discussion of a topic is impossible in a text of this size so, inevitably, the reader will have to read further to get a comprehensive view.

ACKNOWLEDGEMENTS

The illustrations in this text were collected over a number of years by the authors of cases with which they were involved. In many cases the photographer is unknown, and so a general thanks is extended to all the departments of medical photography and illustration with which the authors have worked. A special thanks has to be made for the assistance and permission to reproduce cases of Michael Hawke, Frank Martin, Professor Ian Simson, Professor D.R. Haynes, Dr. M. Lodder, Dr. H. Hamersma and David Smerdon.

The self-portrait of Vincent Van Gogh (p. 51) has been taken from Marc Edo Tralbaut, *Vincent Van Gogh*, Chartwell Books Inc. of 110 Enterprise Avenue, Secaucus, N.J. 07094, 1969.

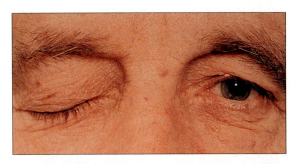

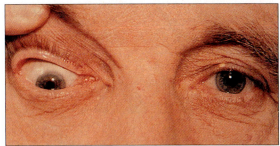

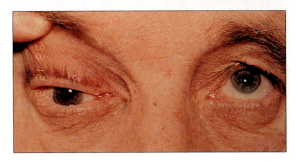

▲ 1

Following relatively minor nasal surgery (sub-mucosal diathermy of the turbinates), this patient awoke from anaesthesia with the right-eye signs illustrated. In the top picture he is gazing ahead; in the second he is raising the eyelid to illustrate the pupil; and in the third he is attempting to gaze upwards.

i. Describe the eye signs.

ii. What other eye movements are tested to isolate the neurological cause?

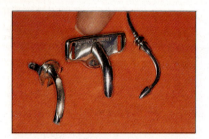

◄ 2

This is an infant tracheostomy tube with associated equipment. Describe the items illustrated and their design features.

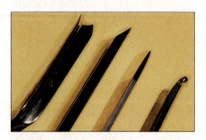

◄ 3

An enthusiastic rhinologist may well take a mallet to these instruments. What are they, and what are their uses?

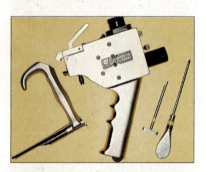

◄ 4

Three of the instruments illustrated may be used in endoscopy. What are their uses and important design features?

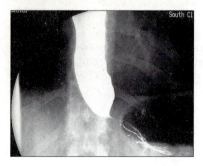

◄ 5

This young man complains of slowly progressive dysphagia with retrosternal discomfort, a tendency to aspiration and weight loss.
i.   What abnormality is revealed on this radiograph?
ii. What is the causative pathology?
iii. What complications may arise?
iv. What treatment is appropriate?

6 ▶

This 50-year-old man presents with a painless upper deep cervical swelling.

i. What radiological technique and characteristic finding is demonstrated here?

ii. What other clinical features should be sought?

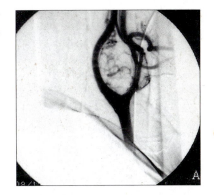

7 ▶

Over a five-year period, an elderly man has noticed slowly enlarging bilateral swelling in the tail of the parotid glands, as shown on this axial CT (computerised tomography) scan.

i. What is the likely underlying pathology and the differential diagnosis?

ii. What investigations may help to confirm the clinical impression?

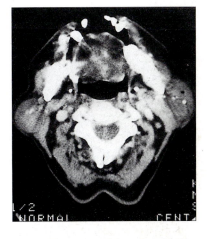

8 ▶

These four instruments might emerge from the distal end of a rigid endoscope in the upper aerodigestive tract. What are they, and what are their uses?

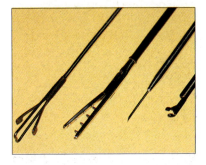

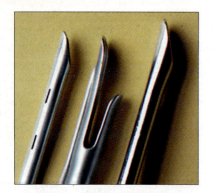

◀ **9**

These three endoscopes can be recognized by their distal ends. What are they?

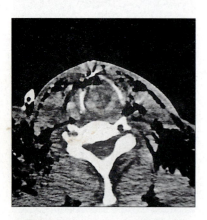

◀ **10**

i. What are the outstanding features of this CT scan of the larynx?

ii. What do these observations indicate?

iii. How should this type of injury be treated?

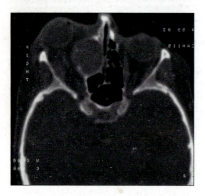

◀ **11**

i. What pathology is demonstrated on this axial CT scan?

ii. What is the differential diagnosis?

iii. What symptoms are likely?

12 ▶

During CT evaluation of a patient with chronic maxillary sinusitis, a mid-line nasopharyngeal lesion was noted and confirmed on mirror examination.

i. What condition is suggested?
ii. What is the differential diagnosis?

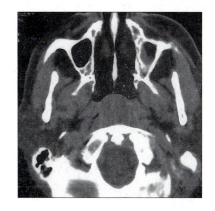

13 ▶

This patient has a long-standing dry perforation of the pars tensa.

i. In an otherwise uncomplicated case, what degree of hearing loss would be expected?
ii. Application of a paper patch in the clinic may produce one of three results: hearing gain; hearing unchanged; hearing worsened. How would you interpret these results?

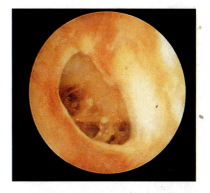

14 ▶

This patient has, for several years, experienced vertigo due to Menière's syndrome and is undergoing surgery for relief. A mastoidectomy has been performed and the antrum has been opened. Further drilling has revealed the cavity in the centre of the picture.

i. What operation is being performed?
ii. What criteria would you apply to patient selection for this procedure?

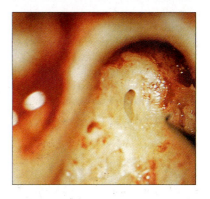

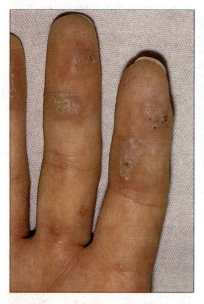
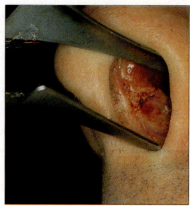

A 40-year-old postman has felt chronically unwell for the past three months. During this period he has experienced a chronic, non-productive cough associated with a bilateral hearing loss, nasal crusting and intermittent epistaxis. Episodically, multiple painful lesions would appear on his fingers, regressing within days (left). Conventional sinus radiographs reveal features compatible with bilateral maxillary sinusitis. Otoscopy confirms the presence of a bilateral serous otitis media. Anterior rhinoscopy demonstrates the lesion shown (right).

i.   What investigations would you request?
ii. A chest radiograph reveals patchy infiltrates to suggest a bilateral bronchopneumonia. Microscopic haematuria is identified on urinalysis. Until proven otherwise, the diagnosis is:
   a. Wegener's granulomatosis;
   b. Churg–Strauss syndrome;
   c. Sjögren syndrome;
   d. Behçet's disease;
   e. Kawasaki disease.

16 ▶

This patient has a unilateral 40 dB air–bone gap and, at tympanotomy, this structure is exposed.

i.   What is revealed?
ii. How may this be managed?
iii. What materials may be used in the surgical management?
iv. Reconstruction succeeds in producing a tenfold gain in delivery of energy to the cochlea. What audiometric gain will result?

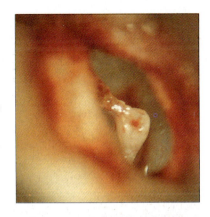

17 ▶

This man presents with left nasal obstruction and this appearance in the oropharynx.

i. What is the diagnosis?
ii. What treatment is indicated?

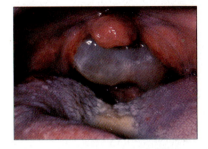

18 ▶

This patient is undergoing exploration of the left maxillary sinus.

i.   What operation is being performed?
ii. What are the indications for this procedure?
iii. What complications may arise?

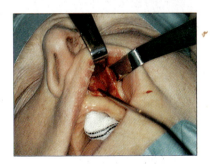

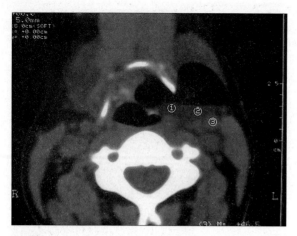

▲ 19

A 60-year-old man presents with a two-year history of an essentially painless, fluctuant swelling in his left anterior neck. Over the previous week he has experienced progressive dysphagia and hoarseness. There has been a long-standing history of cigarette smoking and ethanol abuse. On physical examination a large (5 x 4 cm), non-tender swelling is noted in the left mid-anterior triangle. Laryngoscopy reveals that he has a smooth, non-ulcerated, left-sided swelling. CT imaging demonstrates the abnormality shown above.

i. The diagnosis, until proven otherwise, is compatible with:
    a. combined laryngocele;
    b. branchial cleft cyst;
    c. laryngeal lipoma;
    d. pharyngocele;
    e. Zenker's diverticulum.

ii. This pathology probably arose from an abnormality involving:
    a. the vallecula;
    b. the piriform sinus;
    c. the laryngeal saccule;
    d. the epiglottis;
    e. the upper cervical oesophagus.

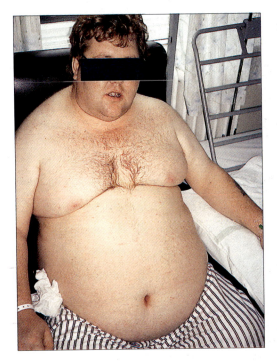

▲ 20

This 45-year-old male is referred for treatment of heroic snoring. From the history, you ascertain that the snoring occurs regardless of what position he sleeps in. Other complaints include daytime lethargy, morning headaches and vivid nightmares. By his own admission, he is 30 kg overweight and hypertensive. On examination, both the palatal tonsils appear moderately enlarged, and he is noted to have bifid uvula. Indirect laryngeal examination is unremarkable and both vocal cords move well.

The most appropriate initial management (investigation and treatment) is:

a. tracheotomy;
b. referral to a weight-loss clinic;
c. uvulopalatopharyngoplasty (UPPP);
d. polysomnogram;
e. prescription for sleeping tablets.

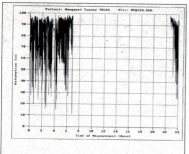

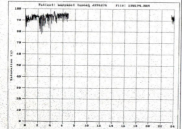

◀ **21**

These tracings represent the results of transcutaneous measurement of oxygen saturation of peripheral blood during sleep before (above) and after (below) therapy.
i. How would you interpret these findings?
ii. What treatment might have produced the second trace?

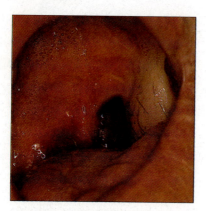

◀ **22**

This man has undergone an extensive resection for a left tonsillar cancer. What appearance is presented here?

23 ▶

This woman has presented with a three-day history of increasing neck pain, a progressive swelling behind the posterior border of the sternomastoid and, now, overlying redness.

i. What is the likely diagnosis?
ii. What complications can develop?
iii. What is the appropriate treatment?

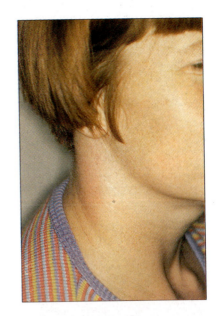

24 ▶

A 12-year-old child has presented with a sore throat of 48 hours' duration; examination reveals this appearance.

i. What is the diagnosis?
ii. How is it confirmed?
iii. What treatment is indicated?

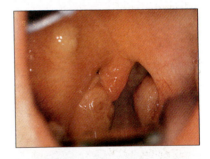

25 ▶

This is an operative photograph illustrating removal of a midline neck swelling to reveal the underlying larynx and trachea.

i. What structures are illustrated?
ii. What is the embryological significance?

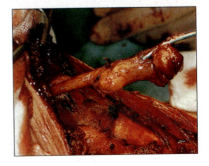

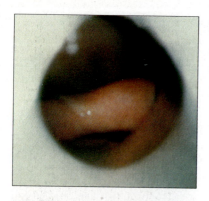

◄ 26

At oesophagoscopy this transverse partition is seen to divide the oesophagus into an anterior and a posterior compartment.

i. What is it?
ii. What operation is being performed during the oesophagoscopy?
iii. Which route leads to the stomach, and which to the law courts?

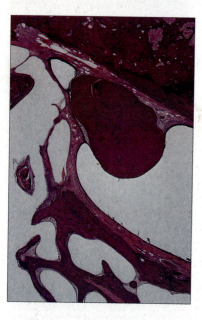

◄ 27

Although asymptomatic while alive, this 70-year-old woman was identified on otoscopy to have a painless solitary swelling in her left external auditory canal (EAC), arising close to the tympanic membrane superiorly. After her death, her temporal bones were harvested and routinely processed. A cross section through the left EAC (stained with H & E) is presented.

The histological diagnosis found in the above illustration is compatible with:

    a. osteoma;
    b. epidermal inclusion cyst;
    c. fibroepithelioma;
    d. ceruminous adenocarcinoma;
    e. sentinel exostosis.

28 ▶

A healthy 40-year-old man presents with a history of recurrent swelling in the left submandibular region. This especially occurs when he eats sour or tart foods. Physical examination reveals a firm, non-tender swelling that involves the left gingival–glossal sulcus posteriorly. The left submandibular gland appears somewhat enlarged as well. A lateral cervical radiograph is shown.

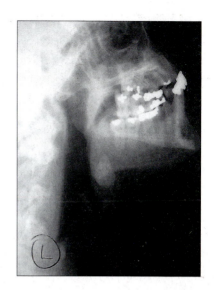

These findings are compatible with:

  a. torus mandibularis;
  b. extensive submandibular sialolithiasis;
  c. plunging ranula;
  d. pleomorphic adenoma of the submandibular gland;
  e. cystic hygroma.

29 ▶

A 55-year-old factory worker presents with a three-month history of a painful, non-healing ulcer involving the under surface of his tongue. Palpable lymphadenopathy is noted in the submental and left submandibular regions. Physical examination reveals the lesion shown here.

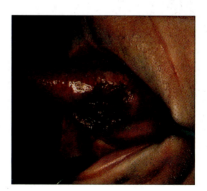

i. Until proven otherwise, this diagnosis represents:
  a. basal-cell carcinoma;
  b. melanoma;
  c. Ludwig's angina;
  d. adenoid cystic carcinoma;
  e. squamous-cell carcinoma.

30

A 25-year-old in her third trimester of pregnancy presents with severe left-sided epistaxis. Conventional anterior and posterior nasal packing is unsuccessful in controlling bleeding. There is no previous history of trauma, and her coagulation parameters are within normal limits. Anterior rhinoscopy reveals no actual bleeding site, but there is a large left-sided inferior nasal spur along the floor of the nose.

i. Appropriate management may include (list as many of the following as are relevant):
    a. septoplasty with formal packing;
    b. selective angiogram with embolization;
    c. stereotactic radiosurgery;
    d. bilateral internal maxillary ligation;
    e. selective angiogram with vasopressin infusion.

ii. The patient undergoes selective angiography with embolization of certain vessels. The vessels that can be typically embolized in the treatment of severe epistaxis are:
    a. the internal maxillary artery;
    b. the facial artery;
    c. the ascending pharyngeal artery;
    d. the anterior ethmoid artery;
    e. the posterior ethmoid artery.

iii. Despite interventional radiological evidence of good embolization by the attending neuroradiologist, the bleeding persists. In this scenario it would be appropriate to ligate both anterior and posterior ethmoid arteries bilaterally.
    a. true;
    b. false.

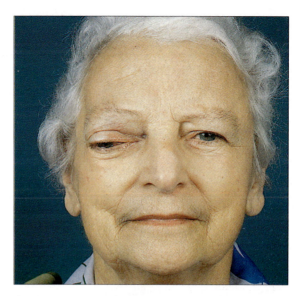

▲ 31

This 75-year-old pensioner presents with a three-month history of right eye pain that has been associated with progressive blindness and proptosis. Her past medical history is unremarkable, although she has been taking thyroid replacement and, two years earlier, had a total abdominal hysterectomy for uterine cancer.

i. In a patient with progressive and painful proptosis, important questions would include:
    a. history of thyroid dysfunction;
    b. previous tumours involving the central nervous system;
    c. previous trauma or surgery to the frontoethmoid sinus complex;
    d. previous ocular surgery;
    e. all of the above.
ii From the case presentation, the least likely cause for her clinical signs and symptoms would be:
    a. Graves' disease;
    b. meningioma;
    c. frontal mucocele;
    d. pseudo-tumour oculi.

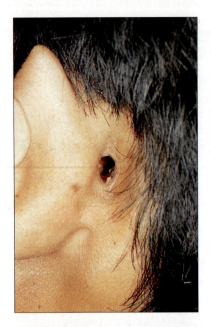

While travelling as a visiting surgeon with the Thai Rural Ear Foundation, you come across an otherwise healthy young man in northern Thailand with a chronic, foul-smelling, left ear. To your surprise, not only are live maggots identified in the ear canal, but there is also a large post-aural fistula.

These clinical findings are most likely to represent:

   a. an extra-pulmonary manifestation of tuberculosis;
   b. the presence of a syphilitic gumma;
   c. a complication of cholesteatoma;
   d. leprosy;
   e. schistosomiasis.

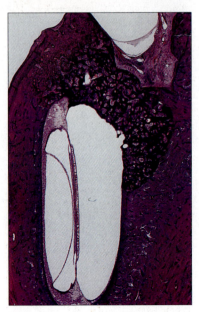

The following cross section (stained with H & E) through the basal turn of the cochlea is taken from a patient who, during her childbearing years, developed a progressive bilateral hearing loss that eventually stopped. Hearing aids provided an appropriate form of aural rehabilitation for her.

The pathologic findings in this illustration are compatible with:

   a. osteopetrosis (marble bone disease);
   b. neurofibromatosis;
   c. Paget's disease;
   d. otosclerosis;
   e. labyrinthitis.

34 ▶

This patient first presented with a transglottic squamous-cell carcinoma of the larynx. He underwent combination treatment with radiotherapy followed by total laryngectomy with good initial result. This is the appearance four months later.

i. What complications have developed?
ii. How may they be avoided?
iii. What treatment is now possible?

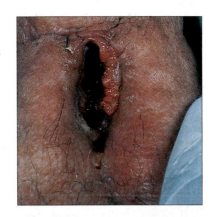

35 ▶

A bright light shone in this man's left eye has failed to produce any reaction, but has caused contraction of the right pupil. When asked to focus on near and far objects alternately, the pupil does dilate and contract.

i. What clinical sign is evident?
ii. What is its relevance to otolaryngology?

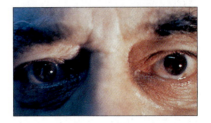

36 ▶

This woman underwent left superficial parotidectomy some months ago but has a post-operative problem during eating.

i. What complication is illustrated?
ii. What treatment is necessary?

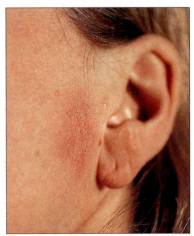

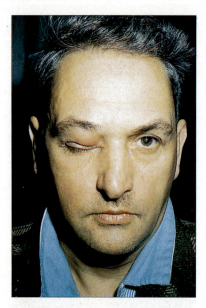

37
This man has developed a minor viral URTI (upper respiratory tract infection), complicated by sudden right frontal headache. He presents the appearance seen here within 24 hours of onset of symptoms.
i. What is the underlying pathology?
ii. What investigations are indicated?
iii. What is the early management?

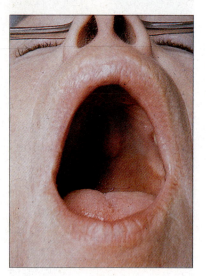

38
This woman recently noticed a midline, painless, hard swelling of the hard palate.
i. What is the likely diagnosis?
ii. What treatment is required?

39 ▶

This 30-year-old man noticed blurring of vision and photophobia with red, painful eyes. Six weeks later he first noticed a left-sided hearing loss with tinnitus and episodic rotatory vertigo. At presentation he now demonstrates the eye signs seen in the photograph.

i. What diagnosis is suggested?
ii. What investigations are needed to establish the differential diagnosis?
iii. What treatment is indicated?

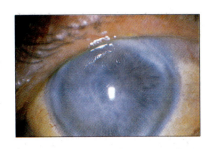

40 ▶

Ophthalmoscopy reveals this appearance at the periphery of a young teenager's visual field.

i. What appearance is presented?
ii. What associated ENT (ear, nose and throat) problems are related to this?

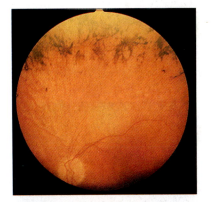

41 ▶

This man initially presented to the neurologist and is now under the care of a head and neck oncologist.

i. What physical signs are demonstrated?
ii. Give three possible causes for the clinical picture presented.

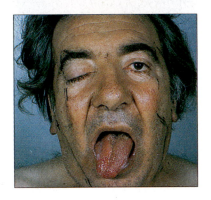

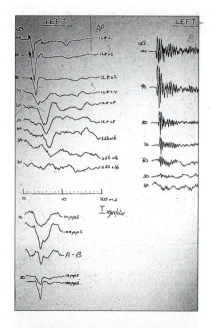

◀ **42**

i. How has this record of cochlear activity been obtained?

ii. What is its clinical use?

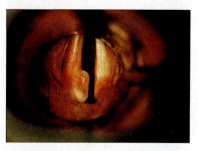

◀ **43**

This photograph has been taken during microlaryngoscopy of a renal transplant patient with hoarseness.

i. What pathology is revealed?

ii. What laryngeal problems are associated with endotracheal intubation, and how are they avoided?

44 ▶

A 12 year-old boy returns from
summer camp complaining of severe
headaches. He has a spiking
temperature and his parents detect a
personality change. A CT scan is
performed, as is shown.

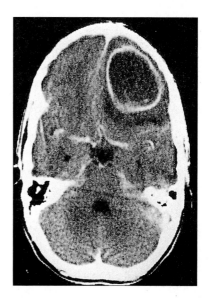

i. The lesion demonstrated in the
   CT scan is:
   a. subdural abscess;
   b. meningitis;
   c. epidural abscess;
   d. parenchymal brain abscess;
   e. sagittal sinus thrombophlebitis.
ii. Two weeks earlier the boy had
    been soldier diving (feet first)
    from a cliff, and this activity was
    associated with the onset of facial
    pain. This complication most
    likely follows a primary infection
    involving the:
    a. frontal sinus;
    b. maxillary sinus;
    c. ethmoid sinus;
    d. sphenoid sinus.

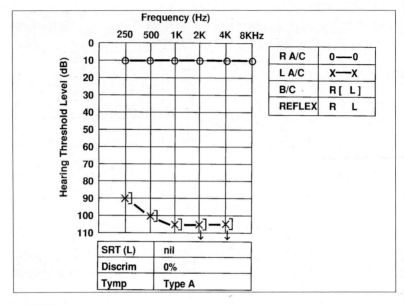

R A/C	0——0
L A/C	X——X
B/C	R [L]
REFLEX	R L

SRT (L)	nil
Discrim	0%
Tymp	Type A

▲ 45

This 50-year-old banker presents within 12 hours of being woken from sleep by a loud hissing sound and complete deafness in his left ear. There has been no associated vertigo or evidence of focal neurological dysfunction. His formal otoneurological examination, apart from a left hearing loss, is unremarkable.

Audiometry reveals the results illustrated.

i. Based on the available information, his diagnosis would be compatible with:
   a. perilymphatic fistula;
   b. sudden sensorineural hearing loss;
   c. Menière's syndrome;
   d. cochlear hydrops;
   e. labyrinthitis.

ii. Six months later the same patient has had no subsequent improvement in either hearing or tinnitus. Appropriate management (investigations/ treatment) might include:
   a. magnetic resonance imaging with gadolinium enhancement (MRI-g);
   b. brainstem-evoked potentials;
   c. conventional hearing aid;
   d. CT scan with enhancement;
   e. contralateral routing of signals (CROS) hearing aid.

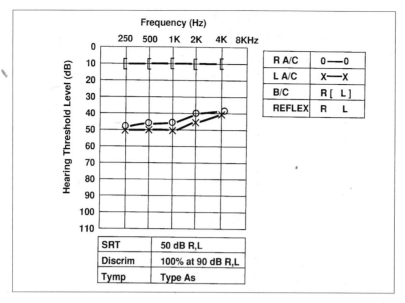

R A/C	0——0	
L A/C	X——X	
B/C	R [L]	
REFLEX	R L	

SRT	50 dB R,L
Discrim	100% at 90 dB R,L
Tymp	Type As

▲ 46

A seven-year-old girl has been documented as having a long-standing, stable hearing loss despite limited improvement from numerous ventilation tube insertions. She currently wears binaural hearing aids which have helped significantly. There is a strong familial history of otosclerosis. Otoscopy reveals her tympanic membranes to be slightly retracted with minimal tympanosclerosis bilaterally. Her audiogram produces the results shown above.

The most probable diagnosis is:

a. recurrent serous otitis media;
b. iatrogenic ossicular dislocation;
c. otosclerosis;
d. congenital malleolar–incus fixation;
e. middle ear tympanosclerosis.

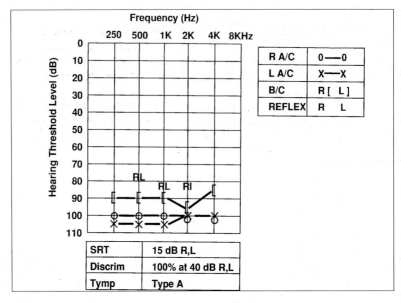

	Frequency (Hz)					
	250	500	1K	2K	4K	8KHz

R A/C	0——0
L A/C	X——X
B/C	R [L]
REFLEX	R L

SRT	15 dB R,L
Discrim	100% at 40 dB R,L
Tymp	Type A

▲ 47

A 50-year-old miner sustained a minor head injury at work which resulted in a transient loss of consciousness. Shortly thereafter, he claims to have become aware of a bilateral hearing loss that has persisted. He has no difficulty in answering your questions. His past otological history has been unremarkable. Otoscopy is normal. Audiometric testing produces the results shown above.

i. Your initial impression suggests that this patient may have:
   a. an unrecognized temporal bone fracture;
   b. an exaggerated hearing loss;
   c. severe noise-induced deafness;
   d. bilateral brainstem coup–countercoup type injury;
   e. central auditory deafness.

ii. Further investigation(s) may include:
   a. repeat audiometry;
   b. cortical evoked-response audiometry;
   c. magnetic resonance imaging (MRI);
   d. high-resolution CT;
   e. central auditory processing tests.

48

A 43-year-old primigravida insulin-dependent diabetic requires an emergency caesarean section for placental abruption. A 31-week gestational female weighing 1,100 g is delivered. Acute resuscitation is required, with transfer to the neonatal intensive care unit (NICU). Three days later, the neonate's condition is complicated by respiratory failure, severe jaundice and the development of Gram-negative sepsis requiring IV (intravenous) gentamicin. Prolonged ventilatory support using increasing concentrations of oxygen unfortunately results in the development of severe retrolental hyperplasia.

i. Factor(s) that place this neonate in a high-risk registry for sensorineural hearing loss include:
   a. advanced maternal age;
   b. placental abruption;
   c. caesarean section;
   d. maternal insulin dependent diabetes;
   e. prematurity;
   f. low birth weight;
   g. Gram-negative sepsis;
   h. oxygen toxicity;
   i. hyper-bilirubinemia;
   j. retrolental hyperplasia.

ii. The baby eventually leaves the NICU, and at six months of age there is strong concern by the mother that her child may have a hearing loss. Appropriate investigations would include:
   a. electroencephalogram (EEG);
   b. behavioural observation audiometry (BOA);
   c. otoemittance testing;
   d. threshold brainstem-evoked potentials;
   e. visual reinforcement audiometry (VRA).

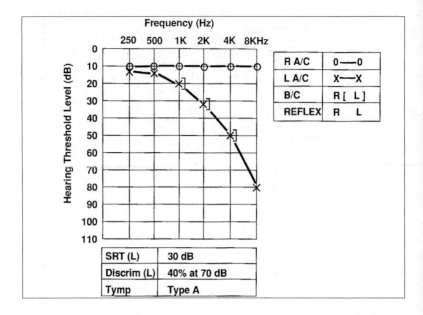

R A/C	0——0	
L A/C	X——X	
B/C	R [L]	
REFLEX	R	L

SRT (L)	30 dB
Discrim (L)	40% at 70 dB
Tymp	Type A

▲ 49

A 30-year-old lawyer has experienced a progressive hearing loss in his left ear over the past year. This has been associated with a constant high-pitched ringing sensation. There has been no fluctuation to hearing, vertigo or evidence of neurological dysfunction. Telephone conversations using the left ear appear garbled and discrimination is difficult, especially in competing background noise situations. Audiometry reveals the results shown above.

If further audiometric testing was required, the most important next test would be:

    a. auditory brainstem response (ABR);

    b. tests for acoustic reflex decay;

    c. cortical evoked-response audiometry (CERA);

    d. performance versus intensity, phonetically balanced (PI–PB) tests;

    e. cortical auditory processing tests (i.e. dichotic, binaural fusion and lower redundancy).

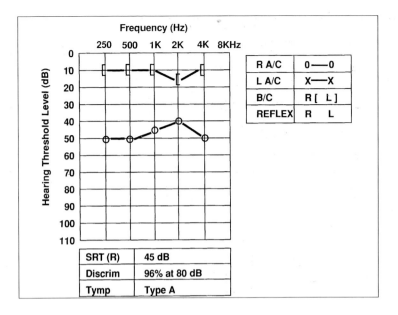

R A/C	0—0
L A/C	X—X
B/C	R [L]
REFLEX	R L

SRT (R)	45 dB
Discrim	96% at 80 dB
Tymp	Type A

▲ 50

For the past three years, a 25-year-old legal secretary has experienced a progressive bilateral hearing loss associated with intermittent tinnitus. The hearing loss appeared to occur during her first pregnancy. Her past otological history has been unremarkable, although her mother experienced a similar hearing loss in her childbearing years. Otoscopy is unremarkable. Her audiogram and impedance measurements are shown above (only the right ear is shown).

i. The most likely diagnosis is:
   a. serous otitis media;
   b. X-linked progressive familial deafness;
   c. otosclerosis;
   d. congenital cholesteatoma;
   e. tympanosclerosis.

ii. The discovery of a reddish hue behind an intact tympanic membrane in this individual would be better known as:
   a. Brown's sign;
   b. Tullio phenomenon;
   c. Hennebert's sign;
   d. Schwartze's sign;
   e. Michael's body.

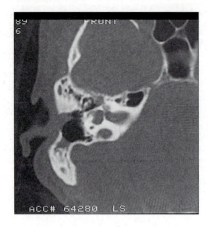

A 23-year-old female has been recently admitted to hospital with her fourth attack of streptococcal pneumonia meningitis following an upper respiratory tract infection. Her past otological history is remarkable for complete deafness in her right ear since childbirth. The right ear has been surgically explored twice, and a posterior fossa craniectomy has also been performed in an attempt to determine a possible portal of entry. Her high-resolution CT axial scan is illustrated here.

Her recurrent meningitis is the result of:

    a. patent cochlear aqueduct syndrome;
    b. Mondini's dysplasia;
    c. a Schiebe–Alexander dysplasia;
    d. congenital mastoid meningo-encephalocele;
    e. Michel's aplasia.

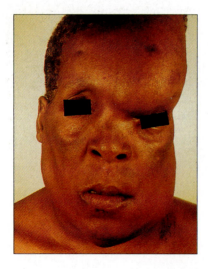

◀ 52

This patient presented to hospital with symptoms relating to a nasopharyngeal carcinoma and not primarily because of the gross deformity due to fibrous dysplasia.

i. Define fibrous dysplasia.
ii. Describe the macroscopic appearance.
iii. What are the microscopic features?

The nasopharyngeal carcinoma is unrelated.

53 ▶

Keratoacanthoma, also known as molluscum sebaceum, is of importance to the otolaryngologist because of its close resemblance to a squamous or basal-cell carcinoma of the skin, e.g. pinna.

i. What is a keratoacanthoma?
ii. What is its macroscopic appearance?
iii. List the histological features.
iv. What are the usual stages in the growth pattern?

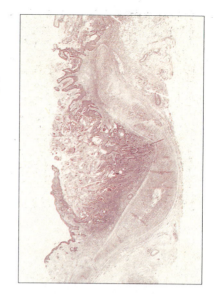

54 ▶

Ameloblastomas are odontogenic tumours of epithelial origin, of which 80% or more occur in the mandible.

i. Name the three clinical types of ameloblastoma.
ii. How does this tumour present in the mandible?
iii. What are the histopathological features?

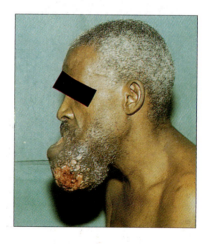

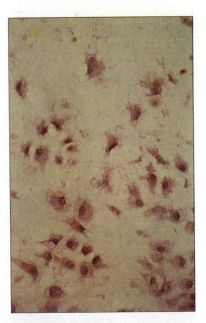

◀ **55**

The chondrosarcoma pictured here was obtained from high up in the nose of a young girl under the age of 10 years. It was initially diagnosed to be a chondroma but, on review, the diagnosis was changed to low-grade chondrosarcoma.

i. Is it a problem to distinguish between a benign chondroma and a malignant chondrosarcoma?

ii. What are the histological indicators of malignancy?

iii. What are the tumours that must be included in the differential diagnosis of cartilaginous neoplasms?

iv. Is chondrosarcoma:
   a. radiosensitive?
   b. responsive to chemotherapy?

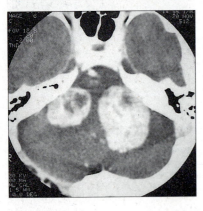

◀ **56**

The abnormalities identified on this enhanced axial CT scan are pathognomonic for:

   a. metastatic renal-cell carcinoma;
   b. neurofibromatosis type 1 (NF1);
   c. neurofibromatosis type 2 (NF2);
   d. congenital epidermoid formation.
   e. chronic subdural haematoma.

57 ▶

The patient illustrated was diagnosed as having squamous-cell carcinoma of the maxillary antrum. The photograph was taken after a full course of radiation therapy.

i. What are the possible complications of radiotherapy?
ii. A soft tissue abscess was drained as indicated by the scars. What are the complications resulting from this surgical intervention?
iii. Why was a maxillectomy not performed in this case?

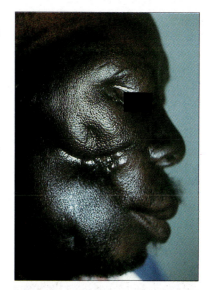

58 ▶

A four-year-old girl is profoundly deaf after meningitis. Her development and speech acquisition were normal until the age of two years, when she became ill. The intra-operative photograph shows a Nucleus 22 implant *in situ* prior to flap closure.

i. What are the indications for a cochlear implant (name at least four)?
ii. List four possible complications of cochlear implantation.

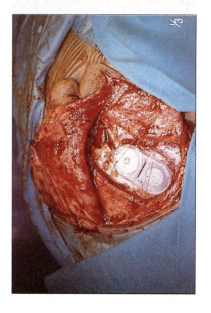

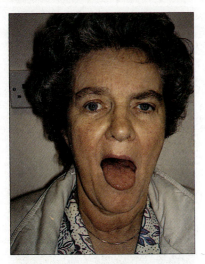

◀ 59

At removal of a large left acoustic neuroma, the facial nerve was cut in this woman. Consequently, she underwent a further operation some weeks later.

What operation has been undertaken?

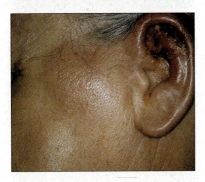

◀ 60

A case of erysipelas is shown with ruptured vesicles on the pinna and the typical streptococcal cellulitis. The latter presents as an hyperaemic, indurated area with clear edges. The involved skin is hot to the touch and is very tender. Regional lymphangitis is common. Bacteraemia with systemic sequelae such as malaise, pyrexia and headache often occur.

i. Make a list depicting the differential diagnosis.

ii. What is the correct treatment?

61 ▶

A basal-cell carcinoma of the medial
aspect of the pinna is presented in
this illustration. It is an example of
malignant neoplasm of the
external ear.

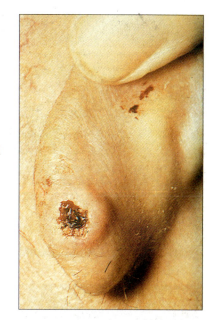

i. Describe the patients most likely
    to develop a basal-cell carcinoma.
ii. What is the biological behaviour
    of this neoplasm, bearing in mind
    that it is also called a 'rodent
    ulcer'?
iii. What percentage of rodent ulcers
    occur:
    a. in the head and neck region?
    b. Of these, what percentage will
       be found on the auricle?
iv. What are the macroscopic
    characteristics?
v. Name the treatment options?
vi. What is the pitfall in the
    treatment?

62 ▶

The illustration is a pre-operative
photograph of a very large keloid of
the post-auricular area, impinging on
the pinna on the right side, after a
previous mastoid operation.

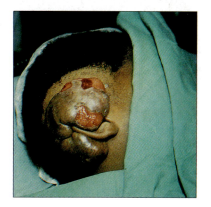

i. Define 'keloid'.
ii. In whom are you most likely to
    expect keloid formation?
iii. Is this condition malignant?
iv. What is the treatment?
v. What is the cause of the keloid in
    this case?
vi. Why is it ulcerating?

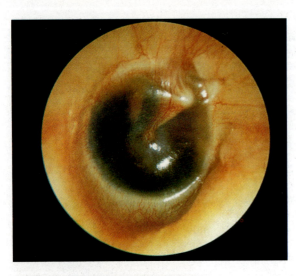

◀ 63

A right-sided tympanic membrane is exhibited showing a dark discoloration in the middle ear.

i. What is the presence of blood in the tympanic cavity called?

ii. What are the causes of this condition?

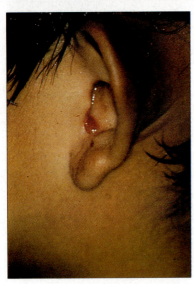

◀ 64

This boy has an acute mastoiditis with a post-auricular abscess. Note the swollen posterior wall of the external ear canal and the purulent discharge. He is clearly flushed, pyrexial and sweaty.

i. What is mastoiditis?

ii. How would you know that an acute middle-ear infection was progressing into an acute mastoiditis?

iii. What are the local signs distinguishing an acute mastoiditis from a furuncle of the external ear canal?

iv. What is the treatment for acute mastoiditis?

65 ▶

A 42-year-old male with a long-standing history of right-sided chronic suppurative otitis media (CSOM) develops a high, spiking temperature (39.5° C) associated with a severe right-sided occipital headache and nuchal rigidity. A previous right mastoidectomy was performed years ago. On examination, he is confused and somewhat lethargic. His gait is ataxic, causing him to fall to the right side. Spontaneous right beating nystagmus is observed. A pulsatile purulent discharge is present in his right ear; the CT scan shows a condition immediately after treatment.

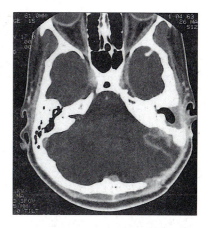

The cause of these symptoms is compatible with:

    a. suppurative labyrinthitis;

    b. petrous apicitis (Gradenigo's syndrome);

    c. cerebellar abscess;

    d. lateral sinus thrombophlebitis;

    e. meningitis.

66 ▶

A very advanced case of lupus vulgaris of the nose and face in a child is presented. The external nose is largely destroyed. Skin, cartilage and mucosa are involved in this patient. Corneal ulceration has taken place.

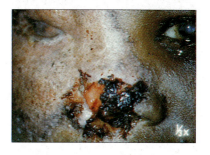

i. What is the aetiology of this condition?

ii. How does the disease present in the early stages?

iii. How should this condition be treated?

iv. What is the differential diagnosis?

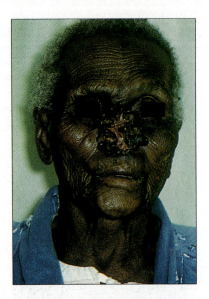

◄ 67

An exophytic mass is seen involving the nose of an elderly woman. The history was relatively short.

i. What are the possible diagnoses (list five)?
ii. How should the diagnosis be confirmed?
iii. What is the correct treatment if the diagnosis is squamous-cell carcinoma?

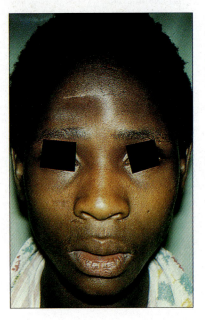

◄ 68

Direct blunt trauma to the forehead resulted in a closed, depressed fracture of the anterior wall of the frontal sinus in this teenager.

i. What are the dangers in this case?
ii. What is the correct treatment in this case where only the anterior wall is involved and where an unacceptable cosmetic defect is present?

69 ▶

A pigmented tumour is shown protruding through the left nostril of this elderly male patient.

i. Make a list of the various ways in which a malignant neoplasm of the nasal cavity may manifest clinically.

ii. Is melanoma of the nose always pigmented?

iii. Are pigmented lesions in the nose necessarily melanomas?

iv. What is the correct treatment, considering that melanomas are radio-resistant and respond poorly to chemotherapy?

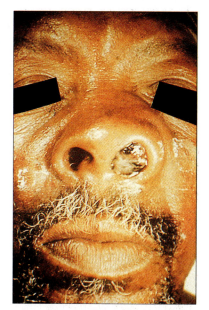

70 ▶

The radiograph presented here is that of a middle-aged woman who suffered from a chronic, unilateral, left-sided maxillary sinusitis.

i. Name three pathological findings pertaining to the maxillary sinus on the radiograph shown.

ii. What are the diagnoses to be considered?

iii. What conditions predispose to the development of aspergillosis?

iv. Name the steps in the treatment.

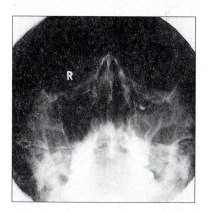

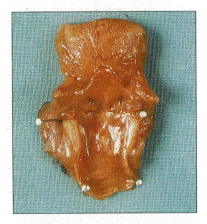

◀ 71

The larynx of a six-day-old pre-mature baby suffering from hyaline membrane disease was examined post mortem to assess the effects of intubation. The child had been intubated shortly after birth using a 3mm Portex nasotracheal tube. This tube was replaced with a 3.5 mm tube on the fourth day. The findings were: 1. Generalized hyperaemia of the larynx; 2. Subglottic ulcerations anterolaterally on both sides.

How could intubation injuries be limited in a neonate?

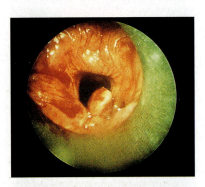

◀ 72

The endoscopic picture shows the subglottic area and upper trachea in a child. Granulation tissue and an inflammatory granuloma are present.
i.   What are the most likely causes?
ii. What are the deleterious effects of this subglottic inflammation?
iii. How should this condition be managed?

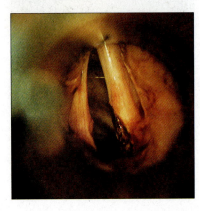

◀ 73

The vocal cord in the illustration has been treated with a laser.
i.   What types of laser are presently used in ENT surgery?
ii. Name eight conditions of the larynx that could be treated with the CO_2 laser.
iii. Why is it better to use the CO_2 laser than other means of removal?
iv. What is a disadvantage of laser surgery from the pathologist's point of view?

74 ▶

In this illustration, hyperaemia of the epiglottis with superficial ulceration and exposure of cartilage is present. The patient was an adult male who complained of very painful swallowing and weight loss. A concomitant infection with *Candida albicans* was present. The primary diagnosis was tuberculosis (TB).

i. What are the clinical features of TB of the larynx?
ii. Which regions of the larynx are most commonly affected?
iii. How should TB of the larynx be treated?

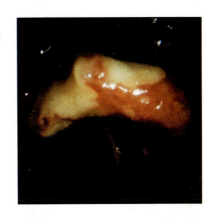

75 ▶

Oedema of the arytenoids, aryepiglottic folds and cords is present and shown in the illustration.

Give a classification of the causes of laryngeal oedema.

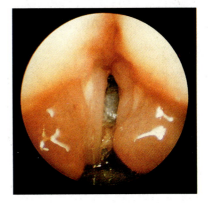

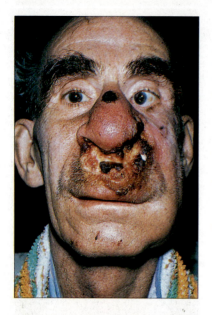

◀ 76

This elderly patient, over a two-month period, has developed a highly destructive lesion of the mid-face, producing ulceration of the upper lip, external nose and nasal septum. A biopsy has been reported as showing acute inflammatory changes only.

i. Outline the investigations required to make a diagnosis.

ii. How does midline granuloma differ from Wegener's granulations?

iii. The diagnosis of midline granuloma is finally confirmed. What is the appropriate treatment and prognosis?

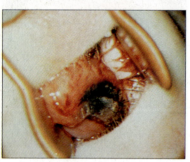

◀ 77

This lesion has arisen on the nasal septum of a young woman.

i. What is the likely diagnosis?

ii. What are the characteristic clinical features of this condition?

78 ▶

This woman hears the tuning fork in her left ear. A previous Rinne test has established that air conduction is better than bone conduction (Rinne positive).

i. What tuning fork test is being used and why?

ii. What is the inference from these test results?

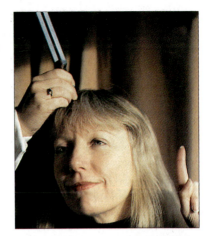

79 ▶

Many years ago, a 60-year-old female had a left mastoidectomy for a chronic draining ear. She is not exactly aware of what happened, but her audiogram demonstrates a maximum conductive hearing loss with a type B tympanogram. Otoscopy reveals the result shown in the illustration.

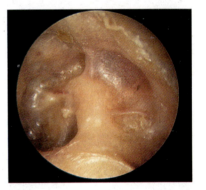

i. The operative procedure most likely performed in the remote past was:

  a. cortical mastoidectomy;

  b. modified radical (Bondy) mastoidectomy;

  c. radical mastoidectomy;

  d. combined approach tympanoplasty;

  e. radical mastoidectomy with mastoid obliteration.

ii. The essential feature(s) of this operation include (list as many as are appropriate):

  a. meatoplasty;

b. an air-containing middle ear space;

c. preservation of the incus or malleus;

d. mastoid cavity;

e. eustachian tube obliteration;

f. lowering of the posterior canal wall to create a common cavity for the middle ear cleft;

g. epithelialization of the entire middle ear with squamous epithelium.

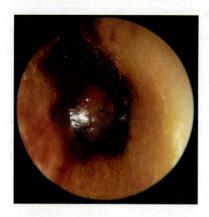

◀ 80

A 35-year-old postman presents with severe otalgia and a serosanguineous discharge from his left ear. His hearing seems to be only slightly diminished. Past medical history reveals that an upper respiratory tract infection occurred approximately one week prior to presentation. The result of otoscopy is illustrated.

i. The most likely diagnosis is:
   a. acute otitis media;
   b. diffuse external otitis;
   c. bullous myringitis;
   d. localized external otitis;
   e. granular myringitis.

ii. The causative organism is often said to be:
   a. *Pseudomonas aeruginosa*;
   b. *Moraxella catarrhalis*;
   c. *Aspergillus niger*;
   d. *Haemophilus influenzae*;
   e. *Mycoplasma pneumoniae*.

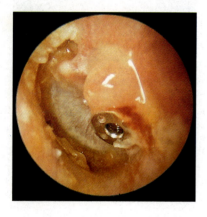

◀ 81

Six months after insertion of a ventilation tube (grommet), this five-year-old child develops an essentially painless purulent discharge from the left ear. Hearing does not appear to be clinically affected. The result of otoscopy is illustrated.

The most likely diagnosis is:
   a. secondary otitis media;
   b. granular myringitis;
   c. secondary fungal external otitis;
   d. implantation cholesteatoma of the middle ear;
   e. tubal granuloma.

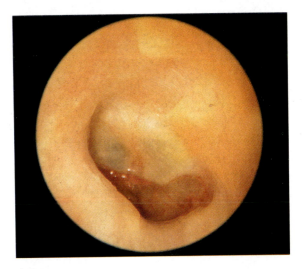

▲ 82

A 41-year-old aircraft pilot has experienced a long-standing history of chronic, intermittent, painless discharge from his left ear. The episodes of discharge usually clear following microdebridement and the instillation of topical antibiotic–steroid drops. Conventional audiometry demonstrates normal pure tone thresholds, and on tympanometry a type A curve is noted. The result of otoscopy is illustrated.

The most likely cause for the intermittent discharge relates to:

    a. granular myringitis;
    b. localized external otitis;
    c. chronic suppurative otitis media (CSOM);
    d. bullous myringitis;
    e. contact dermatitis from the topical antibiotic–steroid drops.

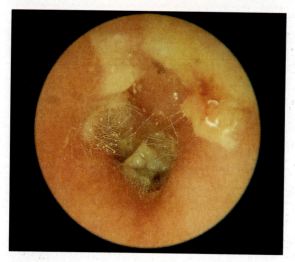

▲ 83

A 20-year-old synchronized swimmer develops a
severely painful left ear and is provisionally diagnosed as
having acute otitis externa (swimmer's ear). Treatment
is instituted with combination antibiotic–steroid drops.
Clinically, the patient seems to improve, only to have a
relapse five days later. This time, although the pain is
not as intense, the ear feels plugged and itchy. The
result of otoscopy is shown in the illustration.

i. The organism most responsible for swimmer's ear is
    Pseudomonas aeruginosa:
    a. true;
    b. false.

ii. Otoscopy now reveals the patient to have:
    a. chronic external otitis;
    b. fungal external otitis;
    c. necrotizing external otitis;
    d. bullous myringitis;
    e. contact dermatitis.

iii. The causative organism in this instance is:
    a. *Staphylococcus aurous*;
    b. *Pseudomonas aeruginosa*;
    c. *Klebsiella pneumoniae*;
    d. *Aspergillus niger*;
    e. *Mycoplasma pneumoniae*.

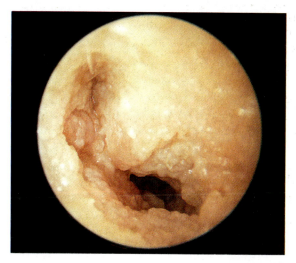

▲ 84

This 70-year-old pensioner has had a long-standing history of chronic left-sided otitis externa. Over the past three months he has become aware of a progressive hearing loss associated with generalized imbalance. Most worrisome, however, has been the recent development of severe otalgia that awakens him from sleep, in conjunction with blood-tinged otorrhea. Although he is in no acute distress when initially examined, it appears that he has a partial left facial palsy.

The clinical history and findings on otoscopy suggest that the most likely diagnosis represents a:

    a. Bell's palsy;
    b. Ramsay–Hunt syndrome (*Herpes zoster oticus*);
    c. complication of cholesteatoma;
    d. glomus jugulare tumour;
    e. carcinoma of the ear canal.

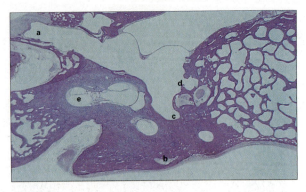

▲ 85

A horizontal cross section of a right temporal bone
(stained with H & E) is provided.

i. Identify the labelled structures a–e.
ii. Anatomically, the sinus tympani extends anteriorly to
   form the eustachian tube:
   a. true;   b. false.
iii. The sinus tympani is an accessible route for combined-
   approach tympanoplasty (CAT):
   a. true;   b. false.
iv. In canal wall-up procedures, recurrent or residual
   cholesteatoma often develops in the sinus tympani:
   a. true;   b. false.

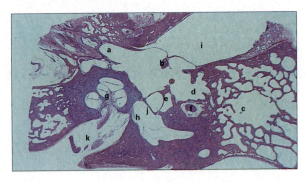

▲ 86

A cross section of this human temporal bone has been
decalcified, sectioned and stained with H & E.

Identify the labelled structures a–k.

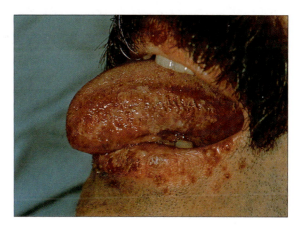

▲ 87

A muscular, 34-year-old man presents with essentially asymptomatic whitish lesions on the lateral aspect of his tongue. Numerous cold sores are also noted on his lower lip.

i. Pertinent questions to ask would include:
   a. risk factors for HIV infection;
   b. smoking history;
   c. recent dental problems;
   d. use of antibiotics and steroids;
   e. all of the above.

ii. The tongue lesions cannot be scraped off. Treatment for oral candidiasis is unsuccessful, so a biopsy is performed. This reveals evidence of hyperkeratosis, parakeratosis and acanthosis of the epithelial layer. The most likely diagnosis is:
   a. Kaposi's sarcoma;
   b. aphthous ulceration;
   c. molluscum contagiosum;
   d. squamous-cell carcinoma;
   e. oral hairy leucoplakia.

iii. In the case of an HIV-seropositive individual, these tongue lesions could be interpreted as a poor prognostic sign:
   a. true;
   b. false.

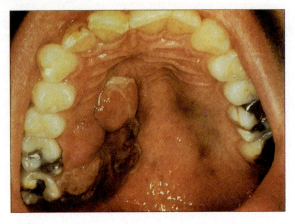

▲ 88

A 38-year-old HIV-seropositive male seeks medical attention for a progressively enlarging, slightly elevated, bluish-coloured lesion on his hard palate. Essentially asymptomatic, it has recently been associated with some intermittent bleeding and ulceration.

i. The most likely diagnosis is:
    a. torus palatini;
    b. Kaposi's sarcoma;
    c. haemangiopericytoma;
    d. pleomorphic adenoma;
    e. non-Hodgkin's lymphoma.

ii. Curiosity kills the cat, so to speak, and it is decided to perform an excisional biopsy for diagnostic purposes. During the procedure, the surgeon receives an inadvertent scalpel blade injury from the knife used in the excision. In this scenario, the risk of occupational HIV seroconversion is best estimated at:
    a. 40%;
    b. 4%;
    c. 0.4%;
    d. 0.04%;
    e. nil.

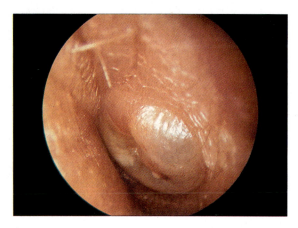

▲ 89

A previously healthy two-year-old child awakens from sleep inconsolable and tugging at his right ear. His mother states that he vomited before bedtime and was slightly irritable during the day. On examination, the child is febrile (39.5°C per rectum) and crying. The result of otoscopy is shown in the illustration.

i. The three most likely causative organisms for this condition, in order, are:
    a. *Moraxella catarrhalis*;
    b. *Pseudomonas aeruginosa*;
    c. *Haemophilus influenzae*;
    d. *Streptococcus pneumoniae*;
    e. *Escherichia coli*.

ii. The child was placed on an appropriate regimen of amoxicillin orally, and sent home. 48 hours later, despite the mother's assurance of compliance, the symptoms and signs appear no better. Likely causes for this include:
    a. gastrointestinal malabsorption of the antibiotics;
    b. the development of a mastoiditis;
    c. presence of beta lactamase-producing organisms;
    d. viral involvement;
    e. presence of cholesteatoma.

iii. In general, beta lactamase-producing organisms are more commonly seen in adults:
    a. true;
    b. false.

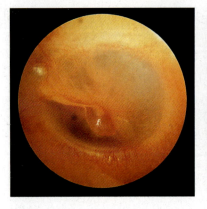 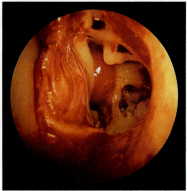

▲ 90

A patient presents with a one-year history of left side tinnitus but no hearing loss. Otoscopy reveals the above findings.

i. What is the likely pathology?

ii. What investigations are necessary to establish the differential diagnosis?

iii. What operation has been performed, and what structures does it reveal?

iv. This lesion displays Brown's sign. What is Brown's sign?

91

A 50-year-old male has had incapacitating attacks of right benign positional paroxysmal vertigo (BPPV) that have followed a head injury. The spells have been present for longer than one year, and he has had no significant periods of remission. Physical examination confirms classic positional nystagmus identified in the Dix–Hallpike (Barany–Nylen) manoeuvre. His hearing appears normal bilaterally.

i. Appropriate medical treatment may include:
   a. physical therapy (liberating or particle repositioning) manoeuvres;
   b. vestibular sedatives;
   c. diuretic therapy;
   d. low-salt diet;
   e. vasodilator therapy.

ii. Should medical treatment fail, appropriate surgical options, considering the suspected pathophysiology of BPPV, would include:
   a. singular neurectomy;
   b. endolymphatic sac decompression surgery;
   c. non-ampullary posterior semicircular canal occlusion;
   d. vestibular neurectomy;
   e. labyrinthectomy.

92 ▶

This temporal bone slide (magnified × 40, stained with H & E) was taken from a patient who experienced episodic attacks of vertigo prior to death. The presence of hearing loss was also documented in that ear.

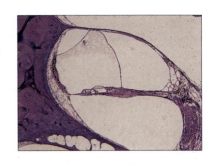

The clinical condition associated with this pathologic finding is:
  a. patent cochlear aqueduct syndrome;
  b. perilymphatic fistula;
  c. labyrinthitis;
  d. recurrent vestibulopathy;
  e. Menière's syndrome.

93 ▶

During his short life, this post-impressionist artist only managed to sell one painting. Today, his works draw the attention of the entire art world and command millions at auctions. His life and the turbulent times surrounding him have been captured in numerous books, movies and popular songs. Why he muti-lated his left ear prior to taking his own life is unknown, but there is speculation that he may have experienced bouts of tinnitus and vertigo.

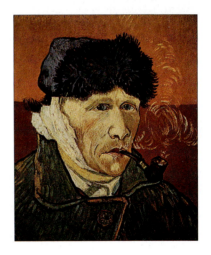

  i. The artist in question is:
      a. Camille Pisarro;
      b. Paul Gaugin;
      c. Vincent van Gogh;
      d. Paul Cézanne;
      e. Edgar Degas.
  ii. The inner ear disorder that this artist may have suffered from is:

  a. otic neurosyphilis;
  b. benign positional paroxysmal vertigo;
  c. perilymphatic fistula;
  d. Cogen's syndrome;
  e. Menière's syndrome.

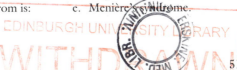
51

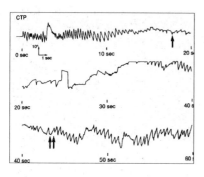

◀ **94**

Prior to commencement of a formal electro-nystagmogram (ENG), a patient complains of severe vertigo while in the caloric test position (CTP). The vestibular technician astutely begins eye movement recordings, and the tracing (left) is obtained in the horizontal leads.

i. Although no clinical history is available at the time, the nystagmus patterns identified have been frequently reported in:
   a. perilymphatic fistula;
   b. labyrinthitis;
   c. otic neurosyphilis;
   d. Menière's syndrome;
   e. benign positional paroxysmal vertigo (BPPV).
ii. From the ENG tracing the most likely involved side is the:
   a. right;
   b. left.

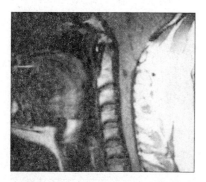

▲ **95**

A 60-year-old female presents with recent complaints of occipital headache made worse with straining, and visual blurring that accompanies head movement. She claims her balance is affected, especially when she looks down. Her past medical history is remarkable for the treatment of tuberculosis with streptomycin 40 years prior. Oculomotor testing demonstrates saccadic pursuit and, in the primary position, spontaneous downbeat nystagmus is identified. A bilateral caloric reduction is noted on formal ENG testing. A magnetic resonance imaging (MRI) scan is illustrated.

The findings are compatible with:
   a. multiple sclerosis;
   b. an Arnold–Chiari malformation;
   c. delayed streptomycin ototoxicity;
   d. atlanto–axial compression;
   e. bilateral Menière's syndrome.

A 60-year-old recluse has experienced progressive growth of a painless ulceration that initially began on her left pinna three years ago. She now seeks medical attention because she finds it difficult to move the left side of her face. On examination you confirm complete left-sided lower motor neurone facial palsy. Tuning fork tests are suggestive of a conductive hearing loss in the left ear.

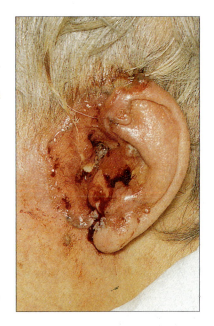

i. The most likely diagnosis is:
    a. squamous-cell carcinoma;
    b. basal-cell carcinoma;
    c. mycosis fungoides;
    d. pyoderma gangrenosum;
    e. keratoacanthoma.

ii. If surgery was contemplated, the most appropriate operative procedure would be:
    a. modified radical mastoidectomy;
    b. radical mastoidectomy;
    c. temporal bone resection with rotational scalp flap repair;
    d. temporal bone resection with local muscle flap rotational repair and a secondary skin graft;
    e. temporal bone resection with a composite myocutaneous flap repair.

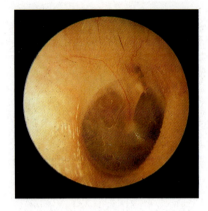

◀ 97

A 42-year-old broadcaster has been aware of a progressive hearing loss in the right ear associated with a vague sense of aural fullness. His past medical history is remarkable for two previous episodes of right-sided idiopathic facial paralysis with incomplete recovery. There is a definite right-sided facial asymmetry present associated with moderate synkinesis. Tuning fork tests were supportive of a conductive hearing loss. The result of otoscopy is shown in the illustration.

The finding of a red mass behind an intact tympanic membrane in the posterior superior quadrant suggests:

    a. acoustic neuroma;
    b. obliterative otosclerosis;
    c. facial nerve schwannoma;
    d. aberrant internal carotid artery;
    e. glomus jugulare tumour.

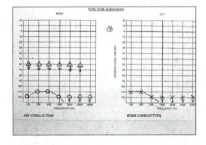

◀ 98

A 45-year-old woman was considered a candidate for a cochlear implant. She gave a 20-year history of progressive hearing loss, initially conductive but with an increasing sensorineural component. There was a strong family history of deafness; her deafness worsened in pregnancy; and, although the diagnosis of otosclerosis was undoubted, poor cochlear reserve prevented stapedectomy. Cochlear otosclerosis worsened until she no longer benefited from a hearing aid.

What surgery could be considered?

99 ▶

i. Why has this woman been into an otolaryngology unit on dozens of occasions and received countless transfusions?

ii. What complications may arise?

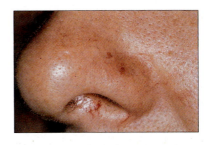

100 ▶

A 14-year-old girl is brought to you by her desperate parents for an expert otological opinion. She has a congenital bilateral hearing loss and failed to develop speech or benefit from any hearing aid. This recently obtained audiogram has raised the hope that surgery might help her. What would you advise?

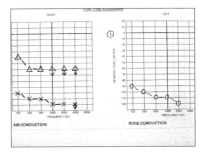

101 ▶

A child suffered a choking episode, with cyanosis, whilst eating, six months prior to presentation. An expiratory wheeze was subsequently noted and attributed to bronchospasm. Failure of bronchodilator therapy led to referral to a paediatrician, who recorded a harsh expiratory sound confined to the left chest with hyper-resonance to percussion.

i. Account for the findings on the chest radiograph.

ii. A bronchoscopy is planned. What anaesthetic hazards does this case present? How may they be avoided?

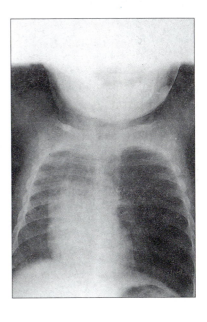

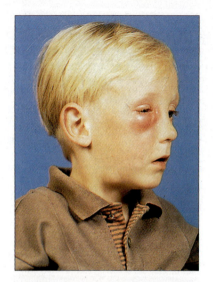

◀ 102

This unfortunate little boy has developed an extremely painful and tender swelling around his right eye over a period of 48 hours. There was no preceding upper respiratory tract infection (URTI), and a sinus radiograph shows a hazy right antrum but no fluid level.

What is the differential diagnosis?

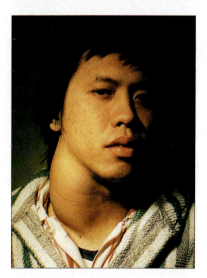

◀ 103

This man has presented with a massive, painless neck swelling, as shown, and a two-month history of epistaxis.

i. What is the likely connection between these symptoms?
ii. What other clinical features should be sought?

104 ▶

Prior to the surgical exploration of a patient with a bulging blue mass behind an intact tympanic membrane, imaging studies are performed. A high-resolution CT scan demonstrates a non-erosive, soft tissue density filling the entire middle ear. On magnetic resonance imaging (MRI), a bright signal intensity is identified on both T1- and T2-weighted images within the middle ear. There is minimal contrast enhancement following gadolinium injection.

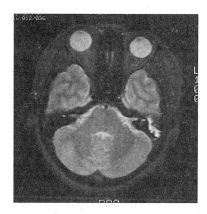

These features are compatible with:
a. aberrant internal carotid artery;
b. glomus jugulare tumour;
c. dehiscent jugular bulb;
d. rhabdomyosarcoma;
e. cholesterol granuloma.

105 ▶

A chondrosarcoma is seen on this CT scan of the larynx. It originated in the cricoid cartilage and enlarged slowly and progressively until it caused obstruction of the airway. Contrast was given but no tumour enhancement occurred. Several initial attempts at biopsy were unsuccessful because the actual tumour was lying deep to calcified cartilage.

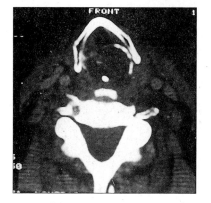

i. Make a list of the characteristics and symptoms of a cartilaginous tumour of the cricoid.
ii. What type of surgery would you have advised in this particular case, and why?

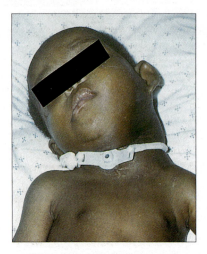

◄ 106

The child shown in the illustration has a marked swelling of his neck on the left side, as well as a distinct scar overlying the mass. His left pinna is displaced anteriorly. The mass caused airway obstruction necessitating a tracheostomy.

i. Write down possible reasons for the neck mass which would lead to a mechanical obstruction of the upper airway.

ii. What are the three categories of indications for a tracheostomy?

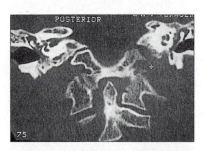

◄ 107

This CT scan was taken of a female patient who presented with a gumma in the nasopharynx.

i. What abnormality do you note?

ii. What stages of the disease can affect bone?

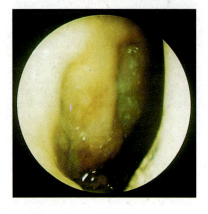

◄ 108

The left eustachian tube orifice is demonstrated showing a syphilitic gumma just proximal to the torus tubarius and involving the fossa of Rosenmüller in the nasopharynx. This is the patient shown in the previous example. The patient also had otosyphilis.

What is the correct medical treatment for otosyphilis?

109 ▶

This man has tuberculoid leprosy.
i. What is leprosy?
ii. What clinical types of leprosy are
    found?

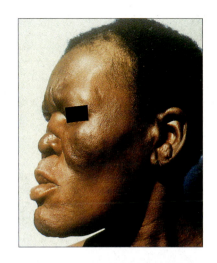

110 ▶

Light-coloured submucosal deposits
are evident on the buccal surface of
the lower lip in this paediatric
patient. The diagnosis is lipoid
proteinosis or hyalinosis cutis et
mucosae. This condition is also
known as Urbach–Wiethe disease.
i. What is the cause of this malady?
ii. How does the abnormality
    manifest?
iii. How should these patients be
    treated?

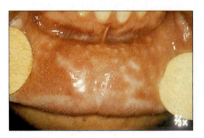

111 ▶

A case of Melkersson–Rosenthal
    syndrome is presented.
i. What are the features of this
    condition?
ii. How should
    Melkersson–Rosenthal syndrome
    be treated?

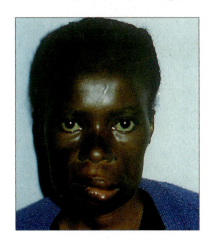

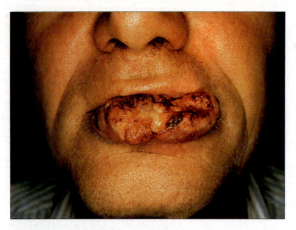

▲ 112

Over the past six months, this 50-year-old grain farmer has developed a progressive, enlarging, fungating mass involving his lower lip. He is quite an avid pipe smoker, and many years ago used to chew oral tobacco. Current medications include prednisone and cyclosporin. These were prescribed following renal transplantation six years ago for treatment of polycystic kidney disease. Palpable lymphadenopathy is noted in the submental and both submandibular regions bilaterally.

i. Until proven otherwise, the most likely diagnosis is:
   a. basal-cell carcinoma;
   b. haemangiopericytoma;
   c. squamous-cell carcinoma;
   d. lymphoma;
   e. widespread actinic keratosis.

ii. Risk factors for the development of this lesion would include all of the following except:
   a. pipe smoking and oral tobacco use;
   b. his occupation as a farmer;
   c. polycystic kidney disease;
   d. prednisone and cyclosporin.

113

What specific investigation should be performed prior to undertaking a blepharoplasty, and why?

114 ▶

A 38-year-old businessman presents with severe right-sided otalgia for the fifth time this year. Treatments with topical antibiotic–steroid drop combinations have always been successful in the past. He denies any history of trauma to the external auditory canal (EAC), and he has not been swimming recently. Otoscopy reveals diffusely swollen EAC, which is extremely sensitive to touch. The tympanic membrane (TM) appears relatively normal following micro-debridement.

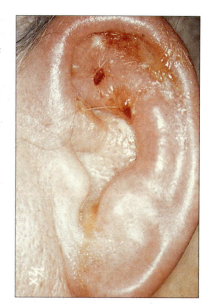

i. The most likely organism responsible for this condition is:
    a. *Moraxella catarrhalis*;
    b. *Streptococcus pneumoniae*;
    c. *Staphylococcus aureus*;
    d. *Pseudomonas aeruginosa*;
    e. *Clostridia difficile*.

ii. Upon further questioning, the patient reveals that he has experienced a slight weight loss and has noticed increasing nocturia. You obviously question whether his otological problem might be a manifestation of a systemic disorder. In this regard, the most likely clinical disorder that needs to be excluded is:
    a. primary hyperparathyroidism;
    b. diabetes mellitus;
    c. Wegener's granulomatosis;
    d. human immunodeficiency virus (HIV) infection;
    e. non-ophthalmic Graves' disease.

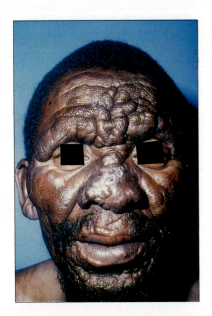

◀ 115
What clinical type of leprosy does this man exhibit?

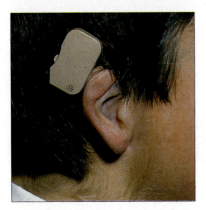

◀ 116
This child has congenital hypoplasia of the external ear.

What does this illustration demonstrate?

A 66-year-old man presents with progressive dyspnoea and inspiratory stridor. His past medical history is remarkable for numerous vertebral compression fractures. Both vocal cords appear mobile, but there seems to be a large, non-ulcerated, posterior subglottic mass. Imaging studies confirm the presence of an expansile mass arising within the framework of the cricoid cartilage. During the course of investigations, the patient is found to be anaemic and to have significant proteinuria. Serum calcium levels are elevated, and an abnormal IgA Kappa paraprotein is identified on immuno-electrophoresis.

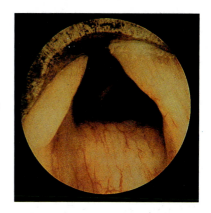

i. The most appropriate investigation(s) prior to a laryngeal biopsy include(s):
   a. bone marrow biopsy;
   b. liver biopsy;
   c. pleural biopsy;
   d. radionuclide skeletal survey;
   e. cystoscopy.

ii Given the clinical history, the most likely diagnosis is:
   a. extra-medullary plasmacytoma;
   b. pan extra-hepatic manifestation of primary biliary cirrhosis;
   c. Wegener's granulomatosis;
   d. multiple myeloma involving the cricoid;
   e. laryngeal lesion associated with a functioning parathyroid adenoma.

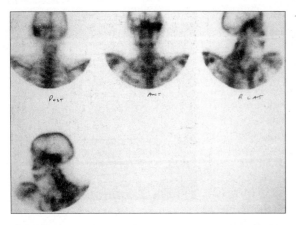

▲ 118

A 50-year-old insulin-dependent diabetic undergoes an uneventful, left-modified radical mastoidectomy in the treatment of cholesteatoma. Three weeks later he is admitted to hospital complaining of severe left-sided otalgia, vertigo and progressive hoarseness. Physical examination reveals a complete left facial paralysis, right-beating spontaneous nystagmus and a paralysed left vocal cord. His mastoid cavity is filled with friable granulations. An urgent technetium-99 scan reveals the results shown.

i. Other important investigations would include all of the following except:
   a. biopsy of granulations for histopathology;
   b. microscopy and culture of discharge;
   c. blood glucose and urinalysis;
   d. high-resolution CT scan of the temporal bone;
   e. carotid angiogram with balloon occlusion/xenon washout test.

ii. The best investigation to confirm whether an infective process is involving the skull base is:
   a. gallium-67 citrate radionuclide scan;
   b. MRI scan;
   c. digital subtraction angiogram;
   d. plain films of the skull base;
   e. air contrast posterior fossa CT scan.

119 ▶

A marked unilateral tonsillar
hypertrophy is to be seen on this
intra-oral view. Note the ulceration
and tendency to bleed on contact.

i. Why is a unilateral tonsillar
   enlargement considered to be
   ominous?

The diagnosis in this instance was a
non-Hodgkin's lymphoma in an
adult.

ii. What are the three grades of non-
    Hodgkin's lymphoma?

iii. What is the treatment in this case,
     which presents only with a uni-
     lateral enlargement of the tonsil?

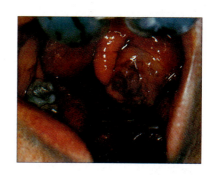

120 ▶

This infiltrate on the upper alveolus
was due to leukaemia.

i. Tabulate the different types of
   leukaemia and the presenting
   ENT symptoms of each.

ii. How is the diagnosis established?

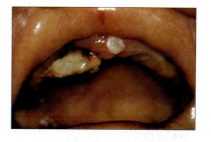

121 ▶

The dorsal surface of this man's
tongue is pigmented and hairy.

i. What is this condition called, and
   what does it signify?

ii. What other colour changes of the
    tongue signify disease?

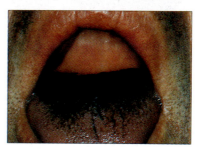

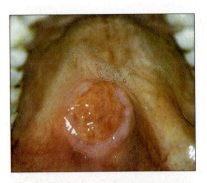

◀ 122
A benign pleomorphic adenoma of the hard palate was diagnosed in this patient.

i. What is the differential diagnosis had she been edentulous and wearing full upper dentures?

ii. Describe the typical clinical presentation of a patient with a pleomorphic adenoma.

iii. What is the correct treatment?

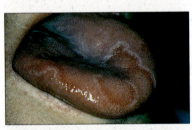

◀ 123
The picture illustrates a geographic tongue.

i. What is the aetiology?

ii. Describe the clinical features.

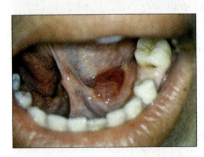

◀ 124
A cystic swelling is present next to the frenulum of the tongue shown here.

i. Name this condition.

ii. What is the underlying pathology?

iii. Describe the treatment.

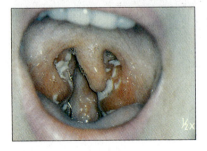

◀ 125
i. What are the systemic symptoms of an acute tonsillitis?

ii. List the local symptoms and signs of tonsillitis.

iii. What type of acute tonsillitis did this patient have, and what other acute type is there?

iv. Name the differential diagnosis.

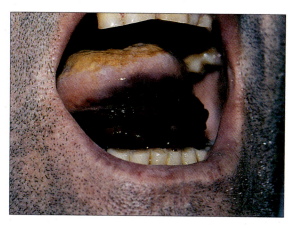

126 ▲

A 50-year-old patient presents with a 24-hour history of progressive stridor and acute dysphagia. He is found to be afebrile and denies any history of recent oral trauma. His past medical history is unremarkable, although he is currently receiving treatment for idiopathic atrial fibrillation with digoxin and coumarin. The result of oral examination is shown.

i.   If this condition was the result of an infection, it would be better known as:
    a. Vincent's angina;
    b. Supraglottis;
    c. Quinsy;
    d. Ludwig's angina;
    e. parapharyngeal abscess.

ii. The most important initial investigation is:
    a. electrocardiogram (ECG);
    b. lateral soft tissue of the neck;
    c. coagulation screen;
    d. high-resolution CT scan of the larynx and pharynx;
    e. panorex of the mandible.

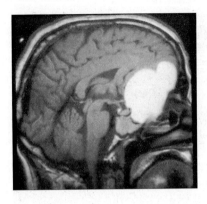

A professional football player sustained an uncomplicated nasoethmoid fracture two years ago. Over the past few months he has experienced dull headaches, and his friends have noted significant changes in his behaviour. An unenhanced magnetic resonance imaging (MRI scan) is shown.

These findings are compatible with a post-traumatic:
  a. mucocele;
  b. caroticocavernous fistula;
  c. olfactory neuroma;
  d. meningoencephalocele.

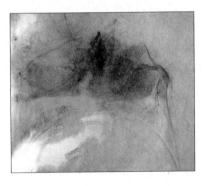

An 18-year-old university student presents with progressive nasal obstruction and significant bouts of apparent posterior epistaxis. Indirect nasopharyngeal examination reveals a bluish mass in his nasopharynx. A selective external carotid angiogram is shown.

i. Until proven otherwise, this lesion represents:
  a. adenoidal hyperplasia;
  b. lymphoma;
  c. cranio-pharyngioma;
  d. sphenoid sinus mucocele;
  e. juvenile nasopharyngeal angiofibroma.

ii A biopsy is necessary to confirm the diagnosis:
  a. true;
  b. false.

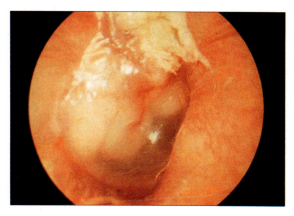

▲ 129

A 16-year-old schoolboy has had a long-standing, painless, foul-smelling discharge from his right ear. Tuning fork tests are suggestive of a right conductive hearing loss. Alternating pressure on his tragus (fistula test) causes him to feel dizzy and produces a few beats of horizontal nystagmus. The illustration shows the result of otoscopy.

i. The most likely diagnosis is:
    a. congenital cholesteatoma;
    b. primary acquired cholesteatoma;
    c. cholesterol granuloma;
    d. rhabdomyosarcoma;
    e. glomus tympanicum.

ii The organism most likely responsible for the foul-smelling discharge is:
    a. *Streptococcus pneumoniae*;
    b. *Aspergillus niger*;
    c. *Pseudomonas aeruginosa*;
    d. *Candida albicans*;
    e. *Moraxella catarrhalis*.

iii A positive fistula test in an individual most probably suggests erosion into the:
    a. cochlea;
    b. endolymphatic duct;
    c. superior semicircular canal;
    d. posterior semicircular canal;
    e. lateral semicircular canal.

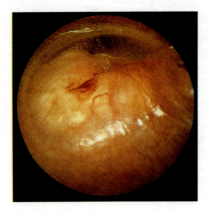

For the past six months this 32-year-old man has been aware of a progressive, painless hearing loss in his right ear. Three years earlier, a simple tympanoplasty was performed using an onlay technique for repair of a safe central tympanic membrane perforation. Tuning fork tests suggest a right conductive hearing loss. Otoscopy reveals a bulging whitish mass behind an intact tympanic membrane.

The most likely diagnosis is:
a. chorda tympani neuroma;
b. implantation cholesteatoma;
c. reactive exostosis;
d. tympanosclerosis;
e. cholesterol granuloma.

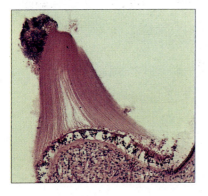

This is a cross section (stained with H & E) through the ampullated end of the posterior semicircular canal.
i. The clinical correlate of this pathologic finding is:
    a. neurofibromatosis type 2 (NF2);
    b. recurrent vestibulopathy;
    c. vestibular neuronitis;
    d. benign positional paroxysmal vertigo (BPPV).
ii. Clinical symptoms that would most likely accompany this pathologic finding include:
    a. continuous, motion-aggravated vertigo lasting weeks;
    b. continuous, motion-aggravated vertigo lasting minutes to hours;
    c. positional-induced vertigo, lasting minutes to hours;
    d. positional-induced vertigo, lasting seconds.

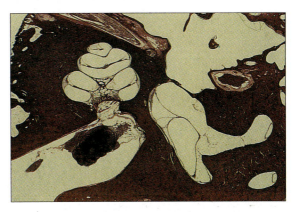

▲ 132

While alive, a 60-year-old electrical engineer was being investigated for a right-sided, unilateral, sensorineural hearing loss. His ENG demonstrated a severe, right-sided caloric reduction in the presence of normal oculomotor function. A high-resolution CT scan was reportedly normal, and no further investigations were performed. At necropsy this temporal bone slide (stained with H & E) was obtained.

The cause for his symptoms was related to:

a. Menière's syndrome;

b. acoustic neuroma;

c. cochlear otosclerosis;

d. meningioma;

e. cupulolithiasis.

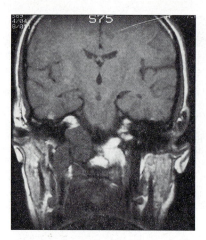

Approximately eight years ago, a benign schwannoma was supposedly totally removed from the left posterior fossa in this patient via a suboccipital approach. The patient did well in the interim, but now returns with a two-year history suggestive of tumour recurrence. His magnetic resonance imaging (MRI) scan is shown.

i. From the location of this tumour in the cerebellopontine (CP) angle, expected left-sided neurological signs might include all of the following except:
    a. diminished corneal reflex;
    b. sensorineural hearing loss;
    c. vocal cord palsy;
    d. fasciculations and hemiatrophy of the tongue;
    e. homonymous hemianopia.
ii. From the MRI scan and the history presented, the two most likely sites for the origin of this tumour are:
    a. the jugular foramen;
    b. the trigeminal nerve;
    c. the hypoglossal foramen;
    d. the facial nerve;
    e. the vestibular nerve.

◀ 134

What procedure is being undertaken here?

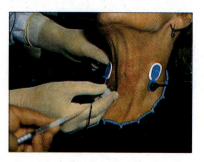

135 ▶

This patient complains of right nasal obstruction.

i. What is the cause?

ii. What is the surgical management available, and what problems are associated with the operation?

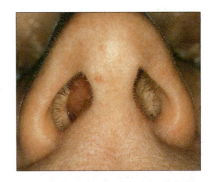

136 ▶

Following dental extraction, this patient notes a foul-smelling nasal discharge and a drainage of pus from the socket.

i. What complication has arisen?

ii. How else may this arise?

iii. What is the management?

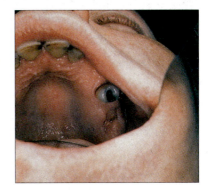

137 ▶

A 50-year-old patient is referred with the illustrated CT scans.

Anterior rhinoscopy reveals a left-sided intranasal mass that is fleshy and pinkish-grey. Following biopsy you are informed that the mass contains a predominance of neurocytes in rosette formations. The most likely diagnosis is:

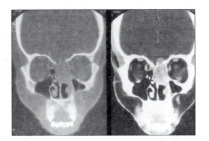

a. inverting papilloma;

b. intranasal;

c. meningoencephalocele;

d. esthesioneuroblastoma;

e. ethmoidal mucocele.

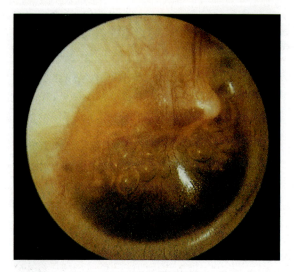

▲ 138

This 30-year-old housewife has experienced a painless hearing loss in her right ear for the past four months, following an upper respiratory tract infection. Indirect nasopharyngeal examination is unremarkable, and otoscopy reveals features similar to the feature illustrated. Tuning fork tests suggest a conductive hearing loss in the right ear.

After much discussion, she consents to a myringotomy and tube (grommet) insertion under local anaesthesia. According to the surgical notes, the procedure was technically difficult and during the myringotomy she developed acute vertigo which lasted for two weeks. When she was reassessed at that time, her audiogram demonstrated a profound sensorineural hearing loss in the right ear.

At a subsequent trial you are asked a number of questions as an expert witness.

i. In your opinion, was the procedure indicated?

    a. yes;

    b. no.

ii. One possible explanation for this unexpected outcome is that it may have occurred if the myringotomy had been performed in a particular quadrant of the tympanic membrane. Which quadrant?

    a. anterior inferior;

    b. anterior superior;

    c. posterior inferior;

    d. posterior superior.

139 ▶

This is the glottis of a child with hoarseness, despite several previous operations.

i. What is the cause of the hoarseness?

ii. What complication has developed as a result of previous treatment?

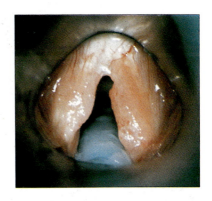

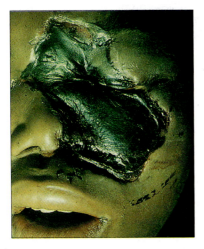

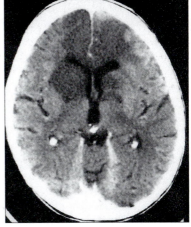

140 ▲

The colour illustration shows a diabetic teenager at the time of his admission to hospital. He was severely ill and in a ketoacidotic coma.

i. What is the condition leading to the clearly demarcated slough of the nose, face and forehead in this patient?

ii. Why does the lesion present in this way?

iii. How should this disease be treated?

iv. Comment on the CT scan of the patient.

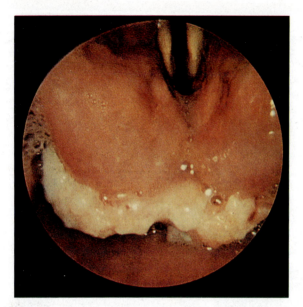

▲ 141

This 55-year-old female has had a long-standing history of iron-deficiency anaemia and chronic dysphagia in the presence of an upper oesophageal web. Despite being a non-smoker, she has recently experienced a progressive hoarseness in her voice and an unintentional 10 kg weight loss. She is concerned because her mother died many years ago from 'throat' cancer. The result of laryngoscopy is illustrated.

i. Until proven otherwise, the provisional diagnosis is:
    a. Zenker's diverticulum;
    b. pharyngeal candidiasis;
    c. post-cricoid carcinoma;
    d. globus hystericus;
    e. chronic hypopharyngeal foreign body.

ii With a more circumspect examination, the presence of atrophic glossitis, angular cheilitis and spooning of the finger nails is identified. When this is taken into account, her diagnosis is most likely compatible with:
    a. Plummer–Vinson syndrome;
    b. Zollinger–Ellison syndrome;
    c. Sjögren syndrome;
    d. Rosenthal–Melkersson syndrome;
    e. avitaminosis C.

142 ▶

Microlaryngoscopy and excision biopsy of the lesion on this man's left cord is reported as 'showing severe dysplasia amounting to carcinoma *in situ* at the anterior resection margin'.

i. What do you understand by this report?
ii. What is the management?

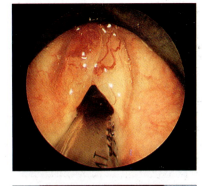

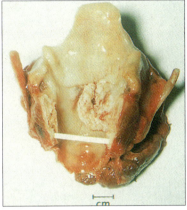

▲ **143**

A total laryngectomy was performed for a squamous-cell carcinoma of the larynx. The lesion involved the ventricular folds and the vocal cords, and extended subglottally for 2.5 cm.

i. What is the TNM classification of the disease in this case, considering that there was no lymphadenopathy or distant metastasis? The right vocal cord was fixed and the thyroid cartilage destroyed at the anterior commissure.
ii. Explain the reasoning for the classification you have selected.

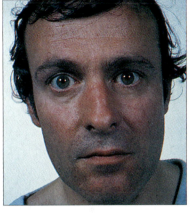

▲ **144**

This man has presented a month after being struck in the left eye by a squash ball. Visual acuity in this eye is unaffected, but he complains of double vision.

i.   What abnormality is demonstrated?
ii. What is the likely cause?
iii. What should be investigated?

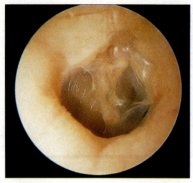

▲ 145

Two years ago, a 25-year-old flagperson sustained a significant closed-head injury when she was inadvertently struck in the right temporal region by a piece of flying metal from a highway road plough. She was transferred to hospital immediately, where loss of consciousness was estimated at approximately 20, minutes and some bleeding was identified from her left ear canal. Shortly after the accident, she became aware of a right-sided hearing loss which has persisted since then, along with attacks of positional dizziness.

When she is assessed in the Dix–Hallpike manoeuvre, no abnormalities are identified in the head-hanging-left position. In the head-hanging-right position, following a latent period of 1–2 seconds, violent geotropic rotatory nystagmus lasting 20–30 seconds is identified. During this time she is vertiginous. When brought upright, the nystagmus assumes an ageotropic reversal that lasts 15 seconds. Repetitive testing causes this response, which is due marginally to fatigue. The result of otoscopy is shown above.

i. The otoscopic finding suggests that she has experienced:
   a. longitudinal temporal bone fracture with an incus dislocation;
   b. longitudinal temporal bone fracture with malleus dislocation;
   c. transverse temporal bone fracture with an incus dislocation;
   d. transverse temporal bone fracture with malleus dislocation.
ii. As an expert witness you are asked by the Compensation Board to provide the diagnosis for her attacks of dizziness. Taking into account her history and the physical findings, her most likely diagnosis is:
   a. perilymphatic fistula;
   b. post-traumatic Menière's syndrome;
   c. post-traumatic atypical positional paroxysmal vertigo;
   d. post-traumatic benign positional paroxysmal vertigo.
iii. The likelihood that these attacks will go into spontaneous remission is:
   a. likely;
   b. unlikely.

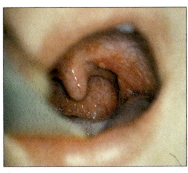

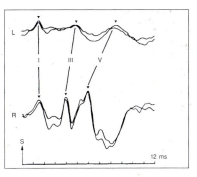

146 ▲

Several mucosal lesions are seen on the anterior faucial pillar and soft palate. They consist of superficial ulcerations surrounded by an area of hyperaemia.

i.   Name a few conditions that could present in this way.
ii. How can Herpes zoster be distinguished from Herpes simplex?
iii. What is the association between herpes and Acquired Immuno-deficiency Syndrome (AIDS)?
iv. How would you treat herpes infection?

147 ▲

The auditory brain stem response pattern (ABR) illustrated here was obtained from a patient with a mild, asymmetric, left-sided sensorineural hearing loss associated with tinnitus.

Appropriate investigation(s) in the future would include:

a. carotid Doppler studies;
b. digital subtraction angiography (DSA);
c. magnetic resonance imaging with gadolinium enhancement (MRI-g);
d. high-resolution enhanced CT scan;
e. radionuclide technetium and gallium imaging.

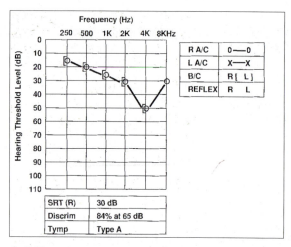

R A/C	0——0	
L A/C	x——x	
B/C	R [L]	
REFLEX	R	L

SRT (R)	30 dB
Discrim	84% at 65 dB
Tymp	Type A

▲ 148

For the past 20 years, this 45-year-old has worked as a jet aircraft mechanic. Recently he has noted a hearing loss, especially in competing background noise situations. His past otological history has been unremarkable, although there is a familial history of deafness with advancing age.

  The result of audiometry of the right ear is shown in the illustration.

  This hearing loss is most likely related to:

a. progressive hereditary deafness;
b. noise-induced deafness;
c. congenital deafness;
d. neurofibromatosis type 2;
e. perilymphatic fistula.

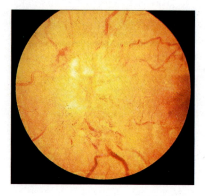

◀ 149

A patient attends the casualty department with a history of confusion and a decreasing level of consciousness. His left ear has been discharging for many years. Examination of the left fundus reveals the result shown here.

i. What does the figure show?
ii. What is the diagnosis, until proven otherwise?

150 ▶

i. What are the obvious abnormalities to be seen in this case?

ii. What is the aetiology of the condition?

iii. What clinical types or stages does the disease manifest?

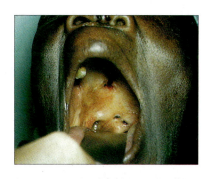

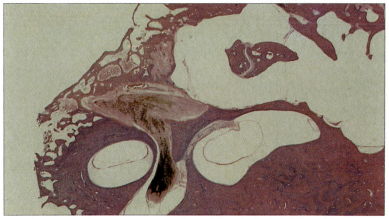

▲ **151**

A 35-year-old male is involved in a fatal motor vehicle accident. Prior to his death, he had experienced a progressive, right-sided facial palsy associated with severe deafness and vertigo in that ear over a three-month period. His past medical history had been essentially unremarkable, apart from the removal of a small pigmented lesion on his back (pathology unknown) three years earlier. A cross section of his temporal bone histopathology (stained with H & E) is shown in the illustration.

Review of the histopathology suggests that the cause of the progressive, right-sided facial paralysis and cochleovestibular loss is secondary to:

a. neurofibromatosis type 1 (NF1);

b. neurofibromatosis type 2 (NF2);

c. metastatic malignant melanoma;

d. metastatic squamous-cell carcinoma;

e. Kaposi's sarcoma.

ANSWER ILLUSTRATIONS

The illustrations below and on pages 84–87 correspond with the answers in the answers section (pages 88–141).

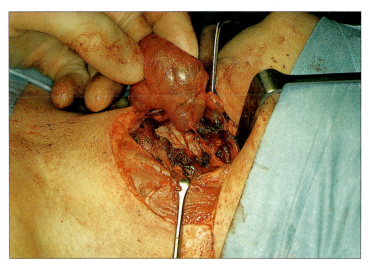

Answer 19 (see page 94).

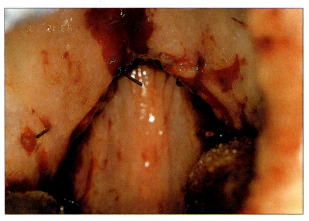

Answer 20 (see page 94).

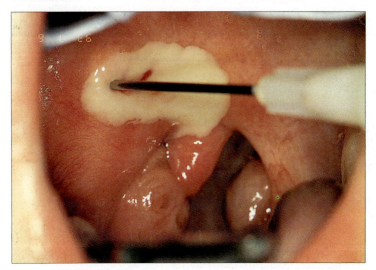

Answer 24 (see page 95).

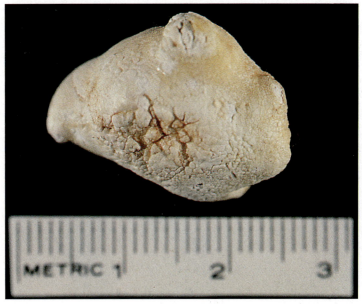

Answer 28 (see page 96).

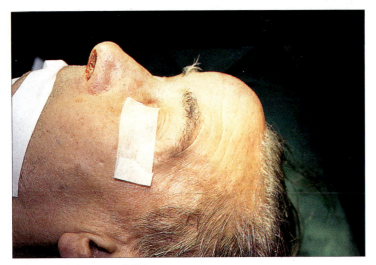

Answer 44 (see page 101).

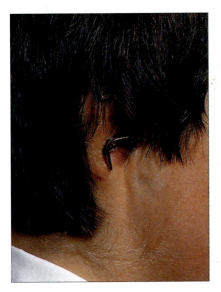

Answer 116 (see page 124).

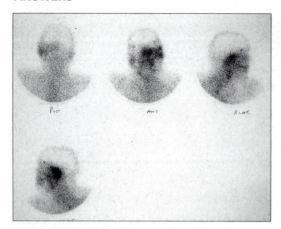

Answer 118 (see page 125).

Answer 126 (see page 128).

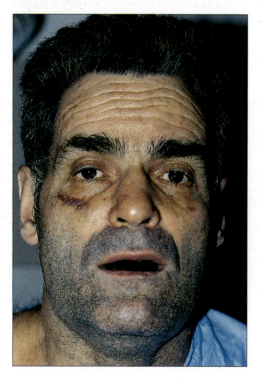

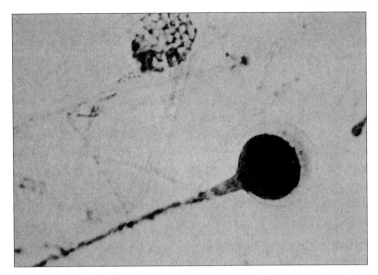

Answer 140 (see page 132).

ANSWERS

1   i. He has a right ptosis and a right ophthalmoplegia, suggesting a III nerve palsy. The pupil is not dilated, so intraocular muscles are spared.

     ii. Lateral gaze should now be tested. If his diplopia is reduced on right lateral gaze, the lateral rectus is functioning and the abducens nerve spared. Downward gaze provides a test of trochlear IV nerve function. Rotation of the pupil on downward gaze suggests IV nerve preservation. This proved to be an isolated III nerve palsy.

         The lack of pupillary involvement is against trauma or posterior communicating artery aneurysm as a cause for this isolated oculomotor lesion. Tumour and uncal herniation are also to be excluded. Medical conditions such as diabetes, atherosclerosis, vasculitis and Guillain–Barré syndrome can produce this isolated cranial neuropathy and spare the pupil.

         A retrograde thrombotic episode was suggested here but fortunately the condition rapidly recovered.

2   The silver tracheostomy tube is inserted using the introducer on the right. The projecting pointed top opens the stomal track to ease entry. On the left is a removable inner tube which prevents occlusion of the tube lumen by dried secretions. This detachable liner is removable for cleaning and replacement with a spare. The inner tube top must project beyond the tracheostomy tube orifice so that no crusting is retained after removal of the inner tube. The flange on the inner tube is notched to allow a lock (not shown) to secure it. The outer tube flange contains two slits to allow insertion of retaining tapes.

         The inner tube illustrated is fenestrated on its upper, convex surface. If combined with a fenestrated outer tube (not shown) it allows inspiration through the tracheostomy but some expiratory flow through the upper airway. This expiratory flow may allow a voice and was considered important for normal growth of the larynx.

3   From left to right these are a gouge, a chisel, an osteotome and a modified osteotome suitable for subcutaneous use.

         The gouge is curved on the flat and is used for rapid removal of chunks of bone. The chisel is bevelled on one surface only and is for shaving a bone surface. The osteotome is bevelled on both surfaces and is designed for splitting a bony plate. The modified osteotome has a notched edge to allow palpation and localization, through the skin of the advancing edge.

4   From left to right these are:
- A laryngoscope. This features a sliding and removable lower plate which has been partly withdrawn. Complete removal allows easy introduction of a bronchoscope through the laryngoscope, which may then be removed.

- A bronchoscope coupler for a CO_2 laser. This handpiece allows delivery of a CO_2 laser beam via a rigid bronchoscope. The articulated arm of the laser attaches to the upper black tube. Sighting is via the black eyepiece on the right, and aiming is helped by the two x–y alignment screws above this. The proximal end of the bronchoscope locks onto the left side of the 'gun'. Below this is a small nozzle which allows delivery of an airflow to prevent fogging of lenses.
- A trochar and cannula designed to puncture the inferior meatus and enter the maxillary antrum. A smaller-bore cannula has long been notorious amongst patients requiring sinus washouts. This trochar is designed to allow passage of sinus endoscopes. The top is bevelled to allow use of right-angled scopes.

5 i. There is a gross dilatation of the thoracic oesophagus, a lack of peristalsis and a failure of the lower oesophageal sphincter to relax. This is the typical appearance of achalasia of the cardia.

   ii. This neuromuscular disorder results from degeneration of the ganglion cells between the circular and longitudinal smooth muscle layers of the oesophagus (Auerbach's plexus). A neurotropic virus may be implicated, and a similar process is found in trypanosomal infection (Chagas' disease).

   iii. The progressive dysphagia leads to malnutrition. Acute distention may cause laryngotracheal airway compression. Chronic retention of undigested food causes oesophagitis, candidiasis and even malignant change. Regurgitation and aspiration may cause recurrent chest infection.

   iv. No treatment can restore peristalsis. The aim instead is to relax or disrupt the lower oesophageal sphincter. Smooth muscle relaxants such as nifedipine or isosorbides may be employed. Pneumatic dilatation and Heller's cardiomyotomy aim to divide the sphincter.

6 i. This is a subtraction carotid angiogram which demonstrates the bifurcation into external and internal branches. The branches are characteristically splayed by the swelling to show the 'Lyre' sign of a carotid body tumour. A later film in the sequence will show the tumour blush.

   ii. The swelling will arise at the bifurcation of the common carotid artery, from the carotid body chemoreceptor. It is generally asymptomatic and spares the adjacent cranial nerves.

   A stethoscope may reveal a bruit, and palpation a thrill. Mobility is present in the anteroposterior plane but absent vertically. An earlier attempt at fine-needle aspiration cytology in this individual filled a 20 ml syringe dramatically!

7 i. The multiple, bilateral, slowly growing parotid mass in an elderly male is very characteristic of a Warthin's tumour (papillary cystadenoma lymphomatosum). It must be distinguished from:
   - intraparotid lymphadenopathy;
   - bilateral pleomorphic adenoma;
   - multicentric parotid cysts with cervical lymphadenopathy in Acquired Immuno-deficiency Syndrome (AIDS).

   ii. MRI of Warthin's tumours demonstrated intermediate signal intensity on T1- and high intensity on T2-weighted images. A Tc–99m scan shows a characteristically high uptake by this tumour, a feature also found in an oncocytoma. Fine-needle aspiration cytology may help, but the majority of parotid neoplasms come to formal excision and histological analysis.

8   From left to right these are:
  - A Clerf Arrowsmith forceps: this is designed to grasp and close an open safety pin to allow safe removal. Success is not easily achieved!
  - A diathermy forceps: used during Dohlmann's procedure, this instrument is used to clamp, crush and coagulate the bar between oesophagus and pharyngeal pouch before final division.
  - This is a shouldered needle for injection of Teflon into a paralysed vocal cord to medialize it and help the opposite cord to achieve glottic closure.
  - A cupped forceps is combined with suction tubing to allow smoke removal during laser microsurgery of the larynx. The blackened surface reduces visible reflection of light and dazzle, but is no protection against CO_2 laser reflection. The deliberately roughened matt surface will scatter the reflected beam, however, and protect against non-target impact.

9   From left to right these are:
  - A bronchoscope. The perforations in the side of the tube are designed to allow escape of anaesthetic gases. Thus, if the bronchoscope is inserted down one main bronchus, gas delivery to the opposite side is maintained.
  - A Dohlmann's oesophageal speculum. This is used to diathermy and divide the partition between an pharyngeal pouch and the oesophagus (and, in doing so, perform cricopharyngeal myotomy).
  - An oesophagoscope. The distal end is bevelled and flared to allow easier inspection and use of forceps.

10   The patient was shot in the face. The bullet fractured the mandible and was deflected downwards through the anterior neck to exit through the larynx.
  i. - A fracture of the thyroid cartilage.
      - Displacement of a portion of the lamina of the cartilage in an anterior direction.
      - Extensive surgical emphysema.
      - An extremely poor residual airway.
  ii. - The wound in the larynx was an exit wound.
       - The airway was violated.
  iii. - Ensure a safe airway by use of tracheostomy.
        - Ensure haemodynamic stability, and treat haemorrhage and shock as indicated.
        - Pain control.
        - Antibiotics.
        - Tetanus toxoid.
        - Direct laryngoscopy.
        - Open exploration and repair.

11   i. There is an expansile lesion of the right ethmoids with thinning, rather than erosion, of the displaced bony margins. It will not enhance and is characteristic of a mucocele.

ii. A malignancy such as carcinoma or lymphoma will erode rather than displace bone. The low-density contents differentiate it from benign soft tissue masses such as inverting papilloma.

iii. There will be a non-axial proptosis and diplopia. Posterior ethmoidal mucoceles can cause cranial neuropathies and mimic nasopharyngeal carcinoma.

12 i. There is a well-circumscribed, low-density, round mass in the mid-line of the posterior wall of the nasopharynx. It proves not to enhance, and mirror examination confirms a blue/brown cystic lesion. This is a congenital Thornwaldt's cyst, a persisting remnant of the pharyngeal bursa which, unless infected, is rarely symptomatic.

ii. A simple mucous retention cyst lies more laterally. Teratomas and dermoids present as polypoid mid-line masses with a heterogeneous radiological appearance due to the varying proportions of ectodermal and mesodermal tissues.

13 i. A simple perforation like this should produce a conductive hearing loss of around 25 dB. An anterior perforation should not expose the round window and compromise the baffle effect. There is tympanosclerosis of the tympanic membrane remnant, and ossicular fixation or erosion would worsen the air–bone gap.

ii. If a paper patch improves hearing, it suggests no major ossicular problem and good prospects for myringoplasty. No hearing gain suggests ossicular fixation by tympanosclerosis. A worsening of hearing suggests ossicular discontinuity. The greatest conductive losses are found when an intact tympanic membrane is associated with disruption of the incudo–stapedial joint.

14 i. This is an osseous labyrinthectomy which has commenced with the opening of the lateral semicircular canal. The operation will continue with exenteration of the posterior and superior canals and removal of neuroepithelium.

ii. This will only be effective in patients with a peripheral vestibular disorder. It is reserved for failure of conservative medical and surgical treatment in the severely vertiginous. As an unselective procedure, hearing is sacrificed. The patient should have a long-standing loss of serviceable hearing with little hope of spontaneous recovery on that side. The opposite ear should show normal hearing and no evidence of any disease process. Elderly patients recover more slowly from the loss of vestibular function.

15 i. • Full blood count (FBC).
• Erythrocyte sedimantation rate (ESR)/Plasma viscosity.
• U & E. Creatinine clearance.
• Mid-stream urine specimen (MSU) – microscopy.
• Plasma protein electrophoresis.
• Chest radiograph. Lung function tests.
• Re-biopsy.
• Antinuclear cytoplasmic antibody.

ii. a. Wegener's granulomatosis.
This uncommon systemic disorder is characterized by the presence of vasculitis and necrotizing granulomas typically involving the lungs and kidneys. Pulmonary

ANSWERS

and renal involvement occurs in 95% and 80% of patients respectively. The renal lesion is typically one of focal necrotizing glomerulonephritis.

Wegener's granulomatosis often presents with symptoms involving the upper respiratory tract, primarily the nose. Early in the disease process it is not unusual to see nasal crusting, epistaxis and rhinorrhea. Chronic sinusitis is said to occur in approximately 90% of patients. The finding of a nasal ulcer is not unusual. The aetiology of Wegener's granulomatosis remains idiopathic. Diagnosis is based on the clinical picture, biopsy results and exclusion of infectious and other granulomatous diseases. Aggressive medical treatment with steroids and immunosuppressive medication (cyclophosphamide, azothiaprine, etc.) is usually recommended. In some patients, treatment with trimethoprim–sulphamethoxazole has been used successfully.

Churg–Strauss syndrome is characterized by the triad of allergic rhinitis, asthma and hypereosinophilia, in association with a systemic vasculitis involving medium and small muscular arteries. Giant-cell arteritis typically involves the temporal arteries and is often associated with jaw claudication, tenderness over the scalp and blindness in nearly one third of untreated patients. Behçet's disease is a vasculitis that usually presents with oral and genital ulcers and uveitis or iritis.

Kawasaki's disease is better known as the mucocutaneous lymph node syndrome. This is characterized by fever, conjunctivitis, red and dry lips, erythema of the oral mucosa, an atypical desquamating rash and cervical lymphadenopathy.

16 i. This shows the stapes head with erosion of the long process of the incus, which is only represented by a fibrous band.

ii. The mobility of the stapes and remaining ossicular chain must be confirmed before repair. Reconstruction of the incudostapedial joint itself is rarely feasible. The incus may be dislocated, removed, drilled to shape and reinserted as an autograft. Incus transposition reconnects the malleus handle to the stapes head.

iii. An autograft, i.e. a graft of the patient's own tissue, is generally favoured. An ossicle shows less tendency to resorption than autologous bone harvested from, for example, mastoid cortex. Cadaver homograft ossicles may be preserved in 70% alcohol or Cialit, but are less popular, due to concerns regarding cross infection. Artificial materials may be bio-inert and not excite a foreign body reaction, or bioactive and bond to bone. Total or partial ossicular replacement prostheses (torps and porps) may be manufactured and drilled to fit. Adhesives based on fibrinogen are increasingly popular in tympanoplasty, but may dissolve bioactive materials.

iv. The decibel rate is logarithmic, so this seemingly good result produces only a 2 dB increase in hearing!

17 i. This is an antrochoanal polyp arising in the maxillary sinus, escaping through the ostium and prolapsing from the middle meatus into the posterior choana.

This lesion is commonest in younger males and is distinct from ethmoidal polyposis. Characteristically, the choanal part resembles the commonest nasal polyps, but lacks eosinophils. A narrow neck often dilates the maxillary ostium and, within the sinus, the connected second lobe of the polyp is often a cyst containing cholesterol-rich fluid.

ii. It is sometimes possible to deliver the polyp *in toto* via traction into the naso-pharynx. Antral puncture drains the cyst, and the cyst wall may be drawn out of the antrum.

The Caldwell–Luc approach ensures complete removal of the antral component but is hazardous to unerupted dentition.

18 i. This is the Caldwell–Luc operation. A sublabial approach to the gingiva buccal sulcus allows an antrotomy to be fashioned in the anterior wall of the maxillary sinus.

ii. This is most commonly performed for treatment of chronic maxillary sinusitis associated with irreversible damage to the antral lining, or for biopsy of an antral neoplasm or removal of an antrochoanal polyp. Infection associated with dental sepsis and oro-antral fistula often requires this approach. A foreign body may be removed from the antral cavity.

Adjacent structures become accessible. A Caldwell–Luc operation provides access to the floor of the orbit for decompression or reduction of a blow-out fracture. Maxillary artery ligation or Vidian neurectomy is performed through the posterior antral wall.

iii. The approach is to be avoided in children due to damage to growth centres, and the upper dentition is always at risk. Closure of the sublabial antrostomy may fail and leave an oro-antral fistula. The infra-orbital nerve may be damaged by excessive retraction.

19 i. a. combined laryngocele.

The clinical and radiological features (which demonstrate an air-containing mass in the neck) are compatible with a combined (external and internal) laryngocele.

By definition, a laryngocele is said to represent a pathologic dilation of the laryngeal saccule, which is found in the laryngeal ventricle (the region between the false and the true vocal cords). With growth, an internal laryngocele expands through weakened areas in the thyro–hyoid membrane (typically where the superior laryngeal nerves have entered into the larynx) and may present as an external swelling in the neck anterior to the sternomastoid muscle. The swelling is classically said to increase during a valsalva manoeuvre and become smaller on palpation. Interestingly, various occupations such as glass blowers, drill instructors, weight-lifters and wind instrument players have supposedly been found to have a higher incidence of this condition. Laryngoceles are often confused with the phenomena of a pharyngocele. There would be different CT findings in patients with a laryngeal lipoma, branchial cleft cyst or Zenker's diverticulum.

ii. c. the laryngeal saccule.

The laryngeal saccule produces mucus which is said to be necessary for vocal cord lubrication. Predisposing factors for laryngocele development include conditions where the saccule is intermittently obstructed (e.g. the so-called ball-valve effect) or where raised intraglottic pressure is forced primarily into the laryngeal ventricle. The development of laryngeal carcinoma in a small number of patients with clinical laryngoceles requires that this sinister condition be excluded prior to surgical removal of the laryngocele. Bryce's sign is a gurgling or hissing sound in the throat that occurs when the external portion of the laryngocele is compressed.

The peroperative appearance of the laryngocele is shown in the illustration on page **83**.

20   d. polysomnogram.

Although snoring is an extremely common phenomenon, the patient's symptoms of daytime lethargy, morning headaches and vivid nightmares require that the condition of sleep apnoea be excluded.

By definition, sleep apnoea represents the cessation of airflow at the level of the nostrils and mouth lasting at least 10 seconds. It is generally agreed that sleep apnoea occurs if at least 30 episodes of apnoea are observed, during both rapid-eye-movement (REM) and non-rapid-eye-movement (non-REM) sleep within a seven-hour sleep period.

A polysomnogram allows for documentation of apnoeic episodes and, during the tests, it is also possible to monitor oxygen saturation via transcutaneous recording electrodes, the electroencephalogram (EEG) response, and the electrocardiogram (ECG). When sleep apnoea is present it is advisable for obese patients to lose weight. In this regard, a formal weight-reducing diet is usually recommended. The use of continuous positive airway pressure (CPAP) has been used as a mechanical approach to prevent pharyngeal airway collapse that seems to occur primarily with the central form of the disease.

UPPP (uvulopalatopharyngoplasty—see illustration on page **83**) is occasionally indicated in patients with obstructive sleep apnoea, although it would be effective in the relief or elimination of snoring in the majority of patients. The presence of a bifid uvula which requires that a submucous palatal cleft be excluded would be a contra-indication to this operation.

A tracheotomy can be a life-saving procedure in patients with severe obstructive sleep apnoea, and it is recommended when there is:
- disabling somnolence;
- life-threatening cardiac arrhythmias during apnoea spells;
- marked oxygen desaturation during sleep;
- no improvement on medical treatment.

If there was evidence that the patient had sleep apnoea, then it would not be recommended to provide a sedative which would aggravate both peripheral and central forms of the disease.

21   i. In the upper trace the patient shows desaturation to levels below 40% on numerous occasions throughout a seven-hour sleep study. Considering the sigmoid shape of the haemoglobin dissociation curve this represents a major physiological insult.

  ii. The lower trace has been achieved by the simple use of CPAP (Continuous Positive Airway Pressure) ventilation. Instead of the lungs passively sucking air into the thorax, a tight-fitting nasal mask allows active ventilation which, pushing air into the upper respiratory tract, acts as a supportive stent. A tracheostomy would have been as effective.

  UPPP is often of benefit in simple snoring, but may be contraindicated in obstructive sleep apnoea as it can compromise CPAP.

22   There is obvious distortion and asymmetry of the soft palate post-operatively. The lateral wall of the oropharynx shows an atypical pallor with, remarkably, hair-growth. Following resection, reconstruction has been accomplished using hair-bearing skin.

      A graft such as this could obtain its blood supply via major cutaneous vessels (an axial flap). This is a composite graft containing skin and bone (a radial forearm flap) revascularized via microvascular anastomosis.

23   i. There is infection of the parapharyngeal or pharyngomaxillary space. This probably represents cellulitis rather than abscess formation, and can arise from tonsillitis, dental disease, perforation of the oesophagus or even mastoiditis.

    ii. Laryngeal oedema may compromise the airway, and infection may involve the neurovascular structures of the neck. Thus, carotid artery erosion, jugular vein thrombophlebitis and cranial neuropathies are all possible.

   iii. Direct spread through the fascial planes of the neck may cause an abscess to point as illustrated. Mediastinitis is a feared complication.

24   i. This is a peritonsillar abscess or quinsy, pointing at the characteristic site.

      The history of a lateralized very sore throat with associated cervical lymphadenopathy is highly suggestive. Inspection is hampered by the marked trismus, but shows peritonsillar swelling, displacement of the tonsil and oedema of the uvula.

    ii. Glandular fever should be excluded, and sophisticated investigations such as ultrasound and CT scanning to distinguish cellulitis from true abscess may be considered.

   iii. In practice, most undergo a trial of aspiration with an 18 FG needle and syringe (see illustration on page **84**), with antibiotic therapy and rehydration. There is little risk of recurrence of an isolated quinsy, and a later tonsillectomy is no longer the rule. In preference, for patients suffering long-standing recurrent tonsillitis, an immediate tonsillectomy is often preferred. Tonsillectomy 'à chaud' is relatively straightforward on the side of the quinsy, but proves a bloody deed on the opposite tonsil!

25   i. This is an operative view of the right side of the anterior neck with the chin on the left. Larynx and trachea are clearly seen. The clamp is holding a cuff of thyroid tissue from the right upper lobe. Beyond the tip of the clamp is a 1–2 cm swelling and a track carefully dissected up to pass beneath the hyoid bone. This is a thyroglossal cyst, with its associated track passing up to the foramen caecum of the tongue.

    ii. The thyroid gland in the foetus arises between the copula and tuberculum impar in the developing tongue, starting at the 17th day of gestation. The primitive gland descends to its adult position through the developing hyoid bone, and may leave a remnant anywhere along this route or indeed never descend and persist as a lingual thyroid. Fistulae are usually due to unsuccessful surgery rather than being congenital.

26   i. This partition divides a hypopharyngeal diverticulum or pouch, posteriorly, from the true oesophageal lumen anteriorly. It contains the circumferential fibres of cricopharyngeus enclosed in mucosa.

ii. This photograph was taken prior to diathermy and division of the pouch, Dohlmann's procedure. Whether by electrocoagulation or CO_2 laser surgery, division of the partition both marsupializes the pouch and performs a myotomy of the upper oesophageal sphincter.

iii. The anterior, oesophageal, lumen can be hard to identify. A vast deep pouch can draw the unwary endoscopist to its fundus and through the wall into the mediastinum. The pouch herniates posteriorly through Killian's dehiscence, in the inferior constrictor.

27　e. sentinel exostosis.

The lesion in the proximal EAC is a sentinel exostosis. Exostoses are localized benign lesions involving the bony EAC that are typically multiple, arise in suture lines near the tympanic membrane and for the most part are asymptomatic. Their aetiopathogenesis is thought to arise from a reactive periostitis that occurs in response to a thermal stimulus and, in the process, is responsible for the deposition of new bone locally. This results in an onion skin–type appearance following decalcification and staining.

Clinically, exostoses are said to be more frequently identified in cold-water swimmers. As the majority of exostoses are asymptomatic, no actual treatment is required. However, when growth obstructs the tympanic membrane, entraps cerumen or causes frequent external otitis, surgical removal is required.

In comparison, an osteoma is a true tumour of bone and typically arises at the bony cartilaginous junction. Histologically, numerous fibrovascular channels are noted, giving the tumour a woven appearance. The remaining possibilities are soft tissue in nature, and would not be compatible with the bony lesion demonstrated.

28　b. extensive submandibular sialolithiasis.

The radiological findings are compatible with a calcified lesion in the left submandibular region. Although a calcified lymph node is a possibility, the most likely cause for this abnormality would be a large submandibular gland/duct calculus. In this patient, an external submandibular gland excision confirmed the presence of a large calculus involving the proximal portion of the submandibular duct (see illustration on page **84**). Calculi are said to occur more frequently in the submandibular duct because the secretions appear to be more viscid. Moreover, there are two sites of anatomic narrowing that involve the submandibular duct (where the lingual nerve crosses its mid portion and at its entrance into the oral cavity), where potential stasis of secretions may allow for the development of the calculi.

29　e. squamous-cell carcinoma.

Basal-cell carcinoma does not occur in this region and it would be unlikely for a mucosal melanoma to present in this fashion. Ludwig's angina represents a rapidly spreading floor-of-mouth cellulitis, and is associated with an enlarged and swollen tongue, not an ulceration. Although an adenoid cystic carcinoma may arise from a minor salivary gland and present with similar findings, it is extremely rare when compared to the prevalence of squamous-cell carcinoma involving the oral cavity.

Risk factors include smoking, oral tobacco use, a history of previous trauma and ethanol abuse.

30 i. a, b & d. Septoplasty with formal packing, selective angiography with embolization and internal maxillary artery ligation.

As this patient's severe, life-threatening epistaxis is persistent, active treatment is required, regardless of the fact that she is pregnant.

In this patient, a large septal spur may actually be hiding a bleeding site and, following its removal, appropriate and firm nasal packing may be placed more easily.

  ii. a, b & c. Both the anterior and posterior ethmoid arteries tend to arise from the internal carotid artery circulation. As a result, these vessels cannot be embolized. This explains why for some patients embolization treatment will fail.

  iii. a. Should bleeding persist then ligation of both anterior and posterior ethmoid arteries may be contemplated. Although the anterior ethmoid arteries are relatively easy to ligate surgically, the same cannot be said for the posterior ethmoid arteries, which are often within 1 cm or less from the optic nerve. In this regard, great care must be taken if an attempt at ligation is made.

31 i. e. all of the above.

In general, the investigation of a patient with unilateral proptosis requires that both local and systemic disorders be excluded. In this regard, investigations are necessary to determine whether pathology involves the frontal sinus (e.g. mucocele), the orbit proper (e.g. a pseudo-tumour oculi) or the anterior cranial skull base (e.g. meningioma with erosion into the orbit). Although Graves' disease (exophthalmos associated with hyperthyroidism) typically involves both eyes, it may occur initially as a unilateral phenomenon. Appropriate imaging studies (conventional sinus radiograph, CT and MRI scans), thyroid function indices and an ophthalmologic assessment are required at minimum.

  ii. a. Graves' disease.

The clinical course of the patient in the case description is least likely to be secondary to Graves' disease. Her imaging studies demonstrated an erosive lesion involving the anterior wall of the frontal sinus with extension into the orbital apex. In fact the clinical presence of a progressive, painful, subacute proptosis associated with blindness was ultimately identified to be secondary to metastatic adenocarcinoma involving the right frontal sinus and orbit. Pathologic correlation confirmed this tumour to be similar to the primary carcinoma that had involved her uterus. This represents an extremely rare site of metastasis for adeno-carcinoma.

32 c. complication of cholesteatoma.

Until proven otherwise, these findings should be taken to be the result of cholesteatoma. Luckily, the patient developed a post-aural fistula in the course of his disease rather than an intracranial complication which could have proven lethal. Maggots, interestingly, tend to keep the ear relatively dry and, in the tropics, this is not necessarily an ominous finding. Although an extrapulmonary manifestation of TB, leprosy and/or a syphilitic gumma in the extreme could also present with these findings, they are definitely rare when compared to the incidence of post-aural fistulae secondary to cholesteatoma. Schistosomiasis would also be unlikely in this regard.

33   d. otosclerosis.

The pathologic finding in this slide demonstrates the so-called 'blue mantle' found in active otosclerosis. Although the term 'otospongiosis' would be a more accurate description of the pathological findings, otosclerosis nevertheless has come to represent a unique disorder that involves the endochondral bone of the human otic capsule.

Otosclerotic foci may arise anywhere in the otic capsule. They consist of an irregular, woven focus of bone that is sharply defined from the otic capsule. When a small focus of otosclerosis does not impair hearing or movement of the stapes footplate, the term 'histologic (non-clinical) otosclerosis' is used. The incidence of so-called histologic otosclerosis is estimated at approximately 10% in various temporal bone series. When the stapes footplate is affected and mobility interfered with, the result is a conductive hearing loss of varying degrees. This is termed 'clinical otosclerosis'. Whether otosclerotic foci can cause a sensorineural hearing loss (cochlear otosclerosis) in the absence of a concomitant conductive hearing loss remains controversial.

34   i. He has a large pharyngocutaneous fistula opening directly into his tracheostomy. Aspiration is an increasing management problem. There is an obvious exophytic mass at the margins of the stoma which proves to be a residual tumour.

    ii. Stomal 'recurrence', which has led to the late wound breakdown, is strictly due to residual disease either in the subglottic mucosa or in paratracheal lymph nodes. It may also be due to tumour implantation if a tracheostomy preceded definitive treatment. Subglottic extension is difficult to gauge clinically and CT scanning or MRI are of benefit. Frozen section analysis of resection margins can indicate residual tracheal tumour. Dissection of paratracheal nodes is easier if the thyroid lobe is sacrificed. A tracheostomy for laryngeal cancer generally demands an urgent laryngectomy with resection of the stoma track.

    iii. At this stage treatment is palliative, aiming to maintain the airway, avoid aspiration and ensure adequate nutrition. At an early stage, stomal excision and manubrial resection allow a lower division of the trachea. Laryngectomy stomas tolerate radiotherapy badly and the prognosis for stomal recurrence is very poor.

35   i. This is an Argyll–Robertson pupil, suggesting neurosyphilis. The pupil does not alter size in response to light, but does so when accommodating. The pupil is characteristically small with irregular margins.

    The contralateral response rules out an afferent pupillary defect (i.e. blindness!). The meiotic pupil of Horner's syndrome does react to light and is associated with ptosis. Such lesions as oculomotor palsy, Holmes–Adie ciliary degeneration, and mydriatic drugs, are associated with pupillary dilatation.

    ii. Syphilis can be manifest in any tissue of interest to the otolaryngologist and may especially mimic malignancy. Neurosyphilis is of special interest in its association with endolymphatic hydrops and Menière's syndrome. Congenital syphilis is, however, a far more significant cause of deafness than acquired tertiary syphilis.

36 i. This is Frey's syndrome. There is post-gustatory sweating and painful flushing over the site of surgery. The pre-auricular portion of the surgical scar is just visible.

Parasympathetic fibres that had stimulated the superficial lobe of the parotid to salivate have regrown into the skin. The stimulus of eating now causes vasodilatation and sweating.

ii. This problem is usually self-limiting. Topical anticholinergic agents such as glycopyrrolate can help, and tympanic neurectomy is employed to denervate the parasympathetic supply. The skin flap can be re-elevated and a fascial graft interposed to prevent further reinnervation.

37 i. He has oedema of the right upper eyelid with no evidence of erythema. Further examination will show extreme tenderness to percussion over the right forehead. His right frontal headache will be worse on coughing or stooping. This is the characteristic picture of frontal sinusitis.

ii. Microbiology of any nasal discharge may ultimately prove helpful. An occipitofrontal plain sinus radiograph may show opacity, or even a fluid level, in the frontal sinus. Clinical examination should seek to exclude ophthalmic or intracranial complications and, if either are suspected, CT or MRI is vital.

iii. The recent onset suggests uncomplicated frontal sinusitis, and treatment aims to sterilize the sinus and restore drainage via the frontonasal duct. Antibiotics and nasal sympathomimetic vasoconstrictors will usually achieve this. A persisting empyema requires frontal sinus trephine. An external incision allows creation of a temporary frontal antrostomy and insertion of a wide-bore drain. This can be removed with restoration of the frontonasal duct patency. A formal fronto-ethmoidectomy is to be avoided during acute sepsis such as this.

38 i. This is likely to be a torus palatinus, a harmless bony swelling of the palatal process of the maxilla. A similar lesion, the torus mandibularis, arises in the inner table of the mandible. Examination will confirm a non-tender, bony, hard swelling with intact mucosa. If it really is of recent origin, however, a salivary tumour is a possibility. Tumours of minor salivary glands show a greater risk of malignancy than those arising in the parotid.

ii. Unless this interferes with fitting of a denture, no treatment is required. Removal is accomplished simply by raising a mucosal flap and removing the prominent bone with a drill.

39 i. The eye demonstrates interstitial keratitis, which, together with symptoms of Menière's syndrome, suggests congenital syphilis or Cogan's syndrome.

ii. Syphilis serology (TPI, FTA, Abs etc.) were all negative in this patient. The diagnosis of Cogan's syndrome is favoured by the almost simultaneous onset of eye and cochleovestibular symptoms in a young patient. This is a systemic vasculitic disease and, for example, aortic valve disease may supervene. The ESR is raised in common with polyarteritis nodosa.

iii. Steroids produce a rapid response if given early, although the prognosis for hearing in most patients is poor.

ANSWERS

40 i. This is what is termed 'bone spicule pigmentation', and is characteristic of retinitis pigmentosa.

  ii. Usher's syndrome is an inherited disorder with a number of minor variants. The usual picture is of a severe congenital deafness with visual problems arising before puberty. Night blindness or field defects add to the auditory handicap. Vestibular involvement with blindness often renders the unfortunate patient ataxic with nystagmus, and anosmia increases the sensory deprivation.

41 i. He has a complete right ptosis and there is no evidence of facial weakness. This implies an oculomotor nerve palsy and, indeed, he has a complete ophthalmoplegia when examined further. On protrusion of the tongue it deviates to the right, suggesting a right hypoglossal nerve paralysis. There are several ink markings on either side of his head, suggesting he is receiving radiotherapy.

  ii. Radiotherapy obviously suggests a malignant process, although a benign inoperable tumour such as a very large glomus jugulare is a possibility. A large tumour is clearly extending from the hypoglossal foramen to the cavernous sinus. A bony secondary deposit, a primary skull base tumour (e.g. osteosarcoma, chondrosarcoma) or extension from a nasopharyngeal tumour could all be implicated.

42 i. This is an electrocochleogram recorded by transtympanic insertion of a needle electrode onto the promontory. 'Near field' recording of cochlear and auditory nerve activity in response to a repeated sound stimulus is detected from background noise by computer averaging.

   The series of tracings on the upper left shows the compound Action Potential. This represents the sum of electrical activity in each fibre of the auditory nerve in response to a series of clicks. The intensity of stimulus is progressively reduced, causing an increasing latency and reduced amplitude of response. The response on the right side shows the cochlear microphonic, a manifestation of hair cell activity in response to sound stimulus.

  ii. The invasive nature of the investigation makes it less popular than BSER (brain-stem-evoked–response audiometry) for threshold examination. It does have two definite advantages, however. It is a very rapidly performed test—the electrical response sought is of a far greater magnitude than that in BSER. It is also free of the masking problem inherent in all other objective audiometry. There is no doubt that the response is solely from the ear under test. In at-risk children undergoing grommet insertion under general anaesthesia, an electrocochleogram (ECochG) gives a useful guide to sensorineural function. It is not frequency-specific, however.

   Radiologic advances and increasingly sophisticated BSER have superseded ECochG in screening for acoustic neuroma. Characteristically, a tumour dramatically widens the action potential and increases the cochlear microphonic.

   Hydrops, as in Menière's syndrome, produces an increased negative summating potential due to distortion of the basilar membrane (see bottom left of ECochG). This finding can provide useful confirmation of the diagnosis in a patient with the characteristic symptoms.

43 i. The patient has an intubation granuloma arising from the vocal process of the arytenoid. Previous endotracheal intubation trauma during prolonged intubation has produced a contact ulcer which went on to granuloma formation and ultimately became a pedunculated polyp.

    ii. During intubation the arytenoid may be dislocated. When intubation is prolonged, a pressure effect with local ischaemia may produce subglottic stenosis or glottic damage, as illustrated. Scarring and even vocal cord paralysis may develop. Ideally, prolonged intubation is to be avoided. Portex tubes are less traumatic than red rubber, and tube movement is avoided. Nasotracheal rather than orotracheal insertion of tubes conforming to the shape of the upper airway is the ideal. A high-volume but low-pressure cuff allows a seal without compromising mucosal circulation.

44 i. d. parenchymal brain abscess.

      The CT scan demonstrates classic evidence of an intracranial parenchymal brain abscess involving the frontal lobe. Enhancement of the tumour capsule is demonstrated following contrast injection. There is evidence of oedema involving the surrounding brain tissue. The pathophysiology of a brain abscess remains controversial, but is thought to arise from retrograde thrombophlebitis involving the veins of the frontal bone and its dural connections. It is relatively unlikely that the abscess arose from a metastatic blood-born dissemination of infection. Both subdural and epidural abscesses would have different characteristics radiologically. Meningitis typically does not present with an abscess formation unless a secondary complication has occurred. Finally, a sagittal sinus thrombophlebitis would demonstrate a central area of infarction along the course of the sagittal sinus.

    ii. a. frontal sinus.

      Frontal sinusitis is relatively rare when compared to involvement of the maxillary and ethmoid sinuses. It is often seen in adolescents, however, especially following trauma to the nasofrontal duct that may occur following activities such as soldier diving. Complications include osteomyelitis of the skull and intra-cranial suppuration (brain abscess, meningitis, subdural abscess, etc.). The presence of a Pott's puffy tumour (see illustration on page **85**) is an interesting clinical condition that often accompanies osteomyelitis of the frontal bone. Multiple subgaleal abscesses are typically identified in areas remote from the osteomyelitis. The individual in the case description underwent frontal trephination and formal drainage of the brain abscess. Long-term antibiotic therapy was required for approximately three months.

45 i. b. sudden sensorineural hearing loss.

      By definition, in the absence of vertigo or a past history of fluctuant hearing loss, a diagnosis of an idiopathic sudden sensorineural hearing loss is most appropriate. Although various mechanisms have been proposed (e.g. viral cochleitis, vascular infarction, etc.), it is virtually impossible in an antemortem investigation to recognise the cause. As a general rule, the natural history of a sudden sensorineural hearing loss is as follows: one third of patients will have normal recovery; another third will recover to an extent; and the latter third will have no improvement whatsoever. In the absence of a recognized cause, treatment is empirical. Bedrest—in combination with intravenous steroids, vasodilator therapy, etc.—has been previously recommended. However, no particular treatment has been able convincingly to demonstrate its efficacy.

 ii. a, d & e. Magnetic resonance imaging with gadolinium enhancement (MRI–g), a CT scan with enhancement and a contralateral routing of signals (CROS) hearing aid.

  As there has been no improvement to hearing or tinnitus over the past six months, the remote possibility that a retrocochlear disorder exists must be excluded. It is estimated that approximately 1% of patients with a sudden sensorineural hearing loss are ultimately found to have an acoustic neuroma. Conversely, 14% of patients with known acoustic neuromas will experience a sudden hearing loss of varying degrees at times.

46 d. congenital malleolar–incus fixation.

  The magnitude of this long-standing, symmetric, bilateral conductive hearing loss in the presence of normal tympanometry would exclude recurrent serous otitis media or an iatrogenic ossicular discontinuity. Otosclerosis rarely presents in children of this age, and more often begins in the late teenage years. Although middle-ear tympanosclerosis causing ossicular fixation is possible, this would also be unlikely in the presence of relatively normal eardrums. The most likely diagnosis therefore is a congenital malleolar–incus fixation in the attic region. When the patient is older, an exploratory tympanotomy would help confirm this diagnosis. A formal ossiculoplasty would more than likely be required to improve hearing.

47 i. b. an exaggerated hearing loss.

  Although the ease of conversation with this individual should have led to suspicion, there is a considerable discrepancy between pure-tone and speech discrimination thresholds. In severe deafness, acoustic reflexes should also never be better than pure-tone thresholds unless an exaggerated response is present. In the absence of a significant head injury or bilateral temporal bone fractures, a brain stem injury is extremely unlikely. As coal mines are generally considered to be quiet compared, for example, to the noise levels identified in hard rock mining, it is unlikely the hearing loss would be occupationally related.

 ii. a. repeat audiometry;
  b. cortical evoked-response audiometry.

  When an exaggerated hearing loss is suspected, it is best to reassure the patient that his/her hearing loss is not as severe as they think. Arrangements can be made for repeat testing which should be performed at least 16 hours after the subject has worked in noise, so as to avoid the phenomenon of a temporary threshold shift (TTS). Although labour intensive, cortical evoked-response audiometry is a useful procedure for confirming accurate threshold measurements, generally within 5–10dB of sincere puretone thresholds.

48 i. b, e, f, g, h & i.

  High-risk factors for neonatal deafness are well established, and these include:
* familial history of childhood hearing impairment;

- congenital perinatal infections (e.g. cytomegalovirus, rubella, herpes, toxo-plasmosis, syphilis);
- anatomical malformations involving the head or neck (e.g. abnormalities of the pinna, overt or submucous cleft palate, dimorphic syndromal or nonsyndromal abnormalities);
- birth weight less than 1,500g;
- hyper-bilirubinemia;
- bacterial meningitis;
- severe asphyxia, which may include those infants with Apgar scores of 0–3 who fail to institute spontaneous respiration by 10 minutes, and those with hypotonia persisting to two hours of age.

Presumably, deafness could also arise from placental abruption (causing intrauterine hypoxia) or, conversely, from oxygen toxicity affecting the developing auditory system as a result of the treatment of this child's respiratory distress syndrome.

ii. c. otoemittance testing;
d. threshold brainstem-evoked potentials.

Kemp's discovery of the cochlear echo has resulted in the development of otoemittance as a diagnostic tool. Ideally suited for neonates and prelingual children, the presence of a cochlear echo indicates that a normal cochlea anatomically, and to a large extent functionally, exists. The cochlear echo, however, may be affected by numerous disorders involving the external auditory canal and middle ear (e.g. serous otitis) and cannot therefore be entirely accurate in the diagnosis of a sensorineural hearing loss.

Multiple threshold brainstem-evoked potentials represent the most accurate means by which to assess the auditory system in infants. There is no role for EEG in the investigation of deafness. BOA may be sensitive to a bilateral severe hearing loss, but its sensitivity and specificity is poor. Visual reinforcement audiometry would be inappropriate, considering this child's visual impairment is a result of retrolental hyperplasia.

49   a. an auditory brain-stem response (ABR).

An asymmetric, unexplained sensorineural hearing loss associated with tinnitus and/or poor speech discrimination requires that a retrocochlear disorder be excluded. The major concern is that the aforementioned patient may have an acoustic neuroma (benign Schwannoma of the vestibular nerve). In this regard, ABR has proven invaluable in the investigation of patients with suspected acoustic neuromas.

In a large, retrospective, series by Bars, Brackman *et al* (1993), 97% of patients with pathologically confirmed acoustic nerve tumours had an abnormal ABR. Although false negatives are rare (i.e. the sensitivity of the test is good), many false positives result (i.e. the specificity may be poor), especially when hearing loss is greater than 75 dB at 4,000Hz.

Historically, both acoustic reflex decay and PI–PB tests were used in the investigation of suspected retrocochlear disorders. Their sensitivity and specificity are poor, however, when compared to ABR. Cortical evoked response tests are primarily useful in the determination of hearing thresholds (e.g. in a malingering patient) and have no active role in acoustic neuroma diagnosis. Tests of central auditory function are not indicated in the investigation of a suspected retrocochlear or cerebellar pontine angle tumour.

50   i. c. otosclerosis;
       ii. d. Schwartze's sign.

Otosclerosis is a unique disorder that only involves the endochondral bone of the otic capsule. This disorder is inherited in an autosomal dominant fashion with incomplete penetrance. The term otospongiosis is often used, and more accurately reflects the pathologic process of new bone formation that primarily involves the stapes footplate, producing a conductive hearing loss. Although there is no sexual predilection in histological otosclerosis, clinical otosclerosis appears to be more common in females and, in some instances, may be exacerbated during pregnancy, suggesting a hormonal link.

Otosclerosis appears bilaterally in 80% of cases, although the degree and progression of hearing loss in the two ears may differ significantly. A Cahart notch (depression in sensorineural hearing at 2,000 Hz) is often seen audiometrically. Controversy exists over whether otosclerosis may in fact cause a concomitant sensorineural hearing loss (the so-called cochlear otosclerosis) in the absence of stapes footplate fixation. Otoscopy is typically unremarkable. Schwartze's sign represents a pink hue arising from the promontory of the middle ear behind an intact tympanic membrane, thought to reflect the deposition of otosclerotic foci.

Treatment may take the form of expectant management, provision of a hearing aid, and/or surgical removal of stapes with insertion of a prosthesis (stapedectomy).

51   b. Mondini's dysplasia.

The radiologic features of this high resolution CT scan are classic for an osseous membraneous abnormality of the labyrinth, better known as Mondini's dysplasia. Key features include an enlarged, dilated, vestibule that is in conjunction with an abnormally thin and probably incomplete plate of bone at the distal end of the internal auditory canal.

In Mondini's dysplasia, CSF leakage and secondary meningitis are two of the more spectacular sequelae. CSF leakage into the middle-ear space is thought to arise in situations causing raised intracranial pressure (e.g. straining, coughing, etc.) exploiting weakness in either the stapes footplate or the membrane of the round window.

Despite two previous exploratory tympanotomies that were associated with obliteration of the footplate region and the round window niche, the patient persisted in having further episodes of meningitis. As a result, a subtotal petrosectomy was performed and the ear canal was closed off in a blind sac fashion according to Fisch. The eustachian tube was defunctioned (thereby isolating the middle ear from the nasopharynx) with autogenous periosteum. The middle-ear cleft was formally obliterated with autogenous fat transferred from the abdomen. To date there have been no recurrent attacks of meningitis.

In Michel's aplasia there is near-complete agenesis of the inner ear. In Schiebe–Alexander dysplasia the osseous portion of the inner ear appears normal radiologically, but there are membraneous abnormalities involving the cochleovestibular neuroepithelium. The patent cochlear aqueduct syndrome is not usually seen in conjunction with a Mondini's dysplasia. There is no evidence radiologically to suggest a mastoid meningoencephalocele.

52 i. Fibrous dysplasia is a benign fibro–osseous condition involving bone. It is mono-stotic or polyostotic. The case in discussion had monostotic fibrous dysplasia involving the frontal bone.

ii. The involved tissue is pale or even white in colour and has the consistency of fibrous tissue rather than bone. Cysts and islands of cartilage may be present. It has a ground–glass appearance on radiograph.

iii. • Thin trabeculae of woven bone in a fibrous stroma.
   • The fibrous stroma is loose and the cells are spindle-shaped.
   • Osteoblasts are conspicuously absent, whereas groups of osteoclasts may be present.

53 i. A localized, non-malignant hyperplasia of squamous epithelium which usually develops on exposed skin. The cause is unknown.

ii. A circular ridge of hyperplastic squamous epithelium surrounding a centrally depressed area containing keratin. The diameter ranges from 1–2 cm.

iii. • Hyperplastic epithelium lying superficially to the sebaceous glands and other skin appendages. Marked acanthosis.
   • A clear transition between the hyperplastic epithelium and normal skin.
   • Surrounding inflammatory reaction with the presence of polymorphs.
   • No dermal invasion.

iv. • Rapid formation over 6–8 weeks.
   • Maturation.
   • Involution lasting 6–8 months or longer.

54 i. • Multicystic intra-osseous.
   • Unicystic intra-osseous.
   • Peripheral soft tissues.

ii. • A slowly progressive, expanding mass.
   • Painless initially.
   • Ulcerates later.
   • Loosens teeth.
   • Interferes with dental occlusion.
   • Size varies from a small tumour to very large growths measuring 10–15cm and more.
   • The majority occur in the posterior region of the mandible.
   • Local infiltration and a very high tendency to recur after removal.

iii. • Ameloblastic epithelium.
   • Fibrous connective tissue.
   • Two patterns exist: follicular and plexiform. The former is more frequently encountered.
   • Cystic areas.

55 i. Intermediate types occur, which makes interpretation difficult. The paucity of mitotic figures in so many chondrosarcomas may be misleading.

   ii. • Pleomorphism.
     • Multinucleated tumour cells.
     • Mitotic figures, but see 55i, above.

   iii • Osteogenic sarcoma.
      • Mixed salivary gland tumours.

   iv. a. & b. No.
     Wide local resection should be performed with close post-operative monitoring for several years.

56 c. neurofibromatosis type 2 (NF2).
    Findings of bilateral, extra-axial enhancing, cerebellar pontine angle masses are classic for neurofibromatosis type 2 (NF2). This disease is decidedly different genetically from neurofibromatosis type 1 (NF1), which is synonymous with Von Recklinghausen's disease or peripheral neurofibromatosis. DNA studies have demonstrated a genetic abnormality on the central long arm of chromosome 22 in NF2 and on chromosome 17 in NF1.

    Approximately 1:50,000 people are afflicted with the NF2 gene. Diagnostic criteria for NF2 have classically required the presence of bilateral acoustic neuromas (or a unilateral acoustic neuroma in an individual with a first degree relative with NF2) and/or the presence of two of the following lesions: meningioma; glioma; Schwannoma; juvenile posterior subcapsular lenticular opacification and neurofibroma. Lesions in NF1 typically produce peripheral neurofibromas and are associated with the presence of café-au-lait spots and Lisch nodules (iris haematomas).

    Both chronic subdural haematomas and congenital epidermoids do not enhance when contrast is given. Although metastatic renal cell carcinoma enhances with CT contrast, it would be unusual for these tumours to arise in both cerebellar pontine angles without significant intra-axial invasion.

57 i. • Hyperpigmentation of the skin.
     • Osteoradionecrosis.
     • Soft-tissue oedema.
     • Soft-tissue necrosis.

   ii. Seeding of carcinoma in the skin can be seen below the scar on his cheek.

   iii. The tumour involves the orbit and parietal region which makes total excision impossible.

58 i. • Profound hearing loss with minimum or no benefit from suitable hearing aid
     • An otherwise healthy person of normal intelligence.
     • Adequate parental and other support.
     • A patent basal turn of the cochlea.

   ii. • Flap necrosis.
     • Post-operative infection.
     • Facial nerve excitation.
     • Dizziness.

59 This patient demonstrates deviation of the tongue to the left with some loss of muscle bulk. She has lost hypoglossal nerve function to the tongue because she has had a XII–VII anastomosis.

60 i. • Acute staphylococcal dermatitis.
  • Perichondritis.
  • Insect bites.
  • Herpes zoster.
  • Angioneurotic oedema.
  • Acute contact dermatitis.
  • Erysipeloid.
ii. • Antipyrexials, e.g. paracetamol
  • Analgesics, e.g. ibuprofen, codeine phosphate
  • Antibiotics (in order of preference):
      Penicillin G/V; Erythromycin; Cephalosporin; Amoxicillin augmented with clavulanate; Clindamycin.

61 i. Fair-skinned persons of either sexes, in the 60–70 age group, who are often exposed to the sun.
ii. It is locally invasive and rarely metastases unless it undergoes change and becomes a squamous-cell carcinoma. The growth rate is slow.
iii. a. 85%
  b. 10%
iv. • Small firm nodule with central dimpling.
  • Later central ulceration with raised edges.
  • At times quite marked covert subcutaneous infiltration into the surrounding tissues.
v. • Wide local excision.
  • Mohs' selective excision.
  • Cryosurgery.
  • Laser surgery.
  • Radiation therapy.
vi. Underestimation and inadequate initial treatment.

62 i. A keloid is an elevated area of scar tissue covered by epidermis, arising at the site of previous trauma.
ii. Young females of Negroid background who have sustained an injury, especially a burn wound.
iii. No.
iv. Treatment is sometimes difficult, with a tendency to recurrence. The options are:
  • Topical or intralesional steroids.
  • Excision.
v. A previous post-auricular incision for mastoid surgery.
vi. Pressure necrosis due to the patient lying on it.

63 i. Haemotympanum.
ii. • Fracture of the temporal bone.
  • Retrograde bleeding into the middle ear via the eustachian tube, e.g. epistaxis.
  • Haemorrhage into the ear from a vascular tumour or arterio-venous anomaly.

ANSWERS

64 i. Mastoiditis is an infection of the mastoid process of the temporal bone involving not only the mucosal lining of the air cells but also the bone itself. It is a complication of otitis media.

ii. The general systemic condition will change in the following ways:
- Malaise.
- Rise in body temperature.
- Erythrocyte sedimentation rate (ESR) increase.
- Leucocytosis with a shift to the left. Otorrhoea becomes mucopurulent and profuse.

iii. • Prior history of middle-ear infection.
- Pressure tenderness over the mastoid.
- Mucopurulent otorrhoea.
- Signs of opacification and osteolysis on radiograph.

iv. • General measures, e.g. pyrexia and pain management.
- Systemic antibiotics.
- Cortical mastoidectomy.

65 c. cerebellar abscess.

Although chronic suppurative otitis media (CSOM) may cause all the listed complications in the question, the radiologic findings and the presence of focal neurological signs/symptoms suggestive of cerebellar dysfunction (right-sided gait ataxia, right-beating spontaneous nystagmus and right occipital headache) point to a right lateral cerebellar abscess.

With regard to the other possibilities, although a suppurative labyrinthitis would be associated with ataxia, a differentiative type nystagmus (left-beating) would have been more likely to be present, and there should be no evidence of focal neurological dysfunction otherwise. Petrous apicitis (Gradenigo's syndrome) by definition requires the presence of severe retro-orbital pain, diplopia and a discharging ear. A lateral sinus thrombophlebitis may be associated with a severe localized pain and a high, spiking temperature, but there should be no evidence of focal neurological dysfunction unless an intracranial complication has arisen. Although meningitis is typically associated with nuchal rigidity, lethargy and confusion, there should be no evidence of focal neurological dysfunction.

Despite previous mastoid surgery, this complication occurred, and a revision mastoidectomy was ultimately required once the intracranial suppuration had settled following neurosurgical drainage and antibiotic therapy.

66 i. Mycobacterium tuberculosis in a patient with relatively high immunity against the disease.

ii. • Vestibulitis.
- Nodule formation.
- Ulceration and granulation.
- Perforation of the nasal septum.
- Scarring and stenosis of the external nose.

iii. Antituberculous medication in children of 6 years of age and younger should consist of the following:
- rifampicin: 10 mg/kg body mass; once daily for 6 months.

- isoniazid: 8–10 mg/kg body mass; once daily for 6 months.
- pyrazinamide: 20–25 mg/kg body mass; once daily for 6 months.
  In addition, calciferol (Vit. D2) should be prescribed.

iv.
- Fungal infection.
- Syphilis.
- Eczema.
- Lupus erythematosus.
- Malignant neoplasms.

67 i.
- Chronic, specific, infective granulomas, e.g. tuberculosis, fungi, syphilis.
- Squamous-cell carcinoma.
- Basal-cell carcinoma.
- Wegener's granulomatosis.
- Lethal mid-line granuloma (lymphoma).

ii. Incision biopsy.

iii.
- Wide local excision.
- Suprahyoid or radical block dissection of neck nodes should they be involved.
- Post-operative radiation therapy if indicated.
- Plastic surgery for cosmetic repair, or glasses-mounted prosthesis.

68 i.
- A covert concomitant fracture of the posterior wall of the sinus with air entrapment in the anterior cranial fossa.
- Cerebrospinal fluid leak into the nose.
- Meningitis.
- Obstruction of the fronto–nasal passage and frontal sinusitis.
- Frontal sinus mucocele or pyocele.

ii.
- Antibiotic cover.
- Elevation of the anterior wall through a limited incision just below the eyebrow.

69 i.
- Nasal obstruction.
- Loss of smell.
- Epistaxis.
- A visible mass.
- Gross local destruction.
- Local and distant metastases.

ii. Amelanotic melanomas are known to occur in the nose, making the diagnosis less obvious.

iii. No. Other pigmented swellings may also be found, e.g.:
- Pigmented basal-cell carcinoma.
- Squamous-cell carcinoma with haemorrhage.
- Septal granuloma.
- Blue naevus.

iv. Wide local excision with primary cosmetic repair.

70 i.
- A very radiodense foreign body. This was in the maxillary antrum, as confirmed by a lateral radiograph.

- Mucosal thickening.
- A fluid level.

ii.
- Aspergillosis due to an infection with *Aspergillus fumigatus.*
- A metallic foreign body.

iii.
- Diabetes mellitus.
- Protracted use of antibiotics.
- Suppressed or inadequate immunity.

iv.
- Surgical removal of the aspergilloma.
- Antifungal treatment, e.g. Amphotericin B, should surgery alone be inadequate.

71
- Atraumatic intubation.
- Avoid unnecessary 'reintubation'.
- Choose the correct sized tube—it should fit comfortably but not too tightly.
- Fix the tube well to avoid movement and abrasion.
- Nasogastric tubes should not be left *in situ* concurrently as this encourages gastric acid reflux.

72 i.
- Prolonged intubation.
- Traumatic intubation.
- Infections, e.g. diphtheria, TB.

ii.
- Acute airway obstruction due to oedema, bleeding or crusting.
- Healing with fibrous tissue formation and the development of a fibrous subglottic stenosis.

iii.
- Appropriate antibiotic cover.
- Adequate humidification.
- Oxygen if necessary.
- Avoid intubation. If the airway is threatened, a tracheostomy should be performed.
- Steroids may be useful short-term if not contraindicated for other reasons.

73 i.
- Carbon dioxide.
- Argon.
- Nd:YAG (neodymium:yttrium aluminium garnet).
- Holmium:YAG.
- KTP 532.
- dye laser.

ii.
- Stenosis, web.
- Papilloma.
- Granuloma.
- Polyps.
- Reinke's oedema.
- Haemangioma.
- Leucoplakia.
- Vocal cord nodules.

iii.
- Haemostasis is readily obtained.
- Excision is accurate.
- Oedema and pain are less.

iv. Tissue that could be used for histology is destroyed by the treatment.

74 i. • Voice changes, e.g. hoarseness or aphonia.
- Dysphagia.
- Submucous infiltration and nodules.
- Ulceration with exposure of cartilage.
- Perichondritis.
- Earache.
ii. • Interarytenoid area.
- Laryngeal aspect of the epiglottis.
iii. • Antituberculous medication in combination, e.g. INH, rifampicin, PAS, ethambutol, streptomycin.
- Adequate nutrition. Surgical intervention should be limited to micro-laryngoscopy and biopsy.
- Family members and close contacts should be examined for possible TB.
- TB is a notifiable disease by law in many countries.

75 • Laryngeal conditions.
- Infections, e.g. acute viral laryngitis, laryngeal diphtheria, tuberculosis, syphilis.
- Trauma, e.g. intubation, penetrating injuries, thermal injuries, corrosives, radiation therapy.
- Foreign body.
- Chronic nonspecific laryngitis, e.g. air pollution.
- Allergic laryngitis.
- Perichondritis.
- Neoplasms.
- Regional pathology, e.g. Ludwig's angina, parapharyngeal abscess, retro-pharyngeal abscess.
- General conditions, e.g. myxoedema, congestive cardiac failure.
  A subglottic stent is in place.

76 i. History and examination should record foreign travel and exclude diabetes and any associated systemic illness.
- MSU: microscopy for haematuria in Wegener's granulations.
- Routine haematology and serum biochemistry.
- Serologic testing for syphilis, fungal disease and anti-neutrophil cytoplasmic antibody (ANCA) for Wegener's granulomatosis.
- CT or MRI scan.
- A further biopsy, sending fresh tissue for immunocytochemistry and 'southern blot analysis', may indicate T-cell lymphoma.
ii. Midline granuloma is a traditional misnomer for a localized reticulosis, i.e. a nasal T-cell lymphoma. Wegener's granulomatosis is a vasculitis with systemic mani-festations. Confusion can arise in lymphomatoid granulations, a peripheral T-cell lymphoma with nasal, pulmonary, cutaneous and neurological lesions. Biopsies of mid-line granuloma may be unhelpful due to the profusion of non-malignant cells (plasma cells, histiocytes, lymphocytes) in the lesion.

ANSWERS

iii. Radiotherapy produces a good initial response. An early recurrence is common and cyclophosphamide and prednisolone may be of benefit. Systemic lymphoma may develop, with a poor prognosis.

77   i. This is a pyogenic granuloma, a nonspecific term applied to granulation tissues arising in response to minor trauma with secondary infection. The lobular capillary haemangioma is a variant of this.

  ii. The painless bleeding polyp can arise on the lip, nasal septum, tongue or oral mucosa, characteristically in females in the 18–40 age group. The lesion may arise in pregnancy and regress spontaneously, and progesterone levels seem to influence vessel size.

78   i. This tuning fork produces a tone of 512 Hz. Tuning forks of lower frequencies can produce vibrotactile sensation, and be felt rather than heard. Higher frequency forks can certainly be heard, but tones decay rapidly and give little time for the patient's observation.

  ii. This Weber test is lateralized to the left and both ears are Rinne positive, tending to exclude conductive loss. The immediate inference is a sensorineural deafness in the right ear. With end organ failure it is obvious that the better ear gives a better response to this bone-conducted stimulus.

However, another possibility arises. This patient may have a conductive deafness in the left, and this is the ear with the worst hearing. We would expect her to be Rinne- negative on this side (bone conduction greater than air conduction) but, in minor degrees of conductive loss, this may not be so. It may take 15–20 dB of air–bone gap to convert a Rinne test to a negative result, but as little at 5–10 dB will lateralize a Weber test to the deafer ear.

The conclusion from these tests in isolation is very limited. There is either a sensorineural loss on the right or a minor conductive loss on the left!

79   i. c. radical mastoidectomy.

  ii. a, d, e, f & g.

Steps involved in a radical mastoidectomy require that an adequate meatoplasty for ventilation and access be provided. In order to create a single squamous epithelial line, non-aerated, middle-ear cavity the eustachian tube is obliterated, the ossicular chain with the exception of the stapes is removed, a mastoidectomy is performed and the posterior canal wall is lowered until it is nearly flush with the vertical segment of the facial nerve.

80   i. c. bullous myringitis

Bullous myringitis is an acute inflammatory disorder that clinically involves the tympanic membrane (TM) and the external canal wall skin. It is characterized by a severe otalgia and the presence of blood-filled haemorrhagic vesicles involving the TM. When the vesicles rupture a serosanguinous discharge is often seen. In comparison to acute otitis media, bullous myringitis is typically associated with only a mild conductive hearing loss. Some patients, however, have shown symptoms suggestive of cochlear involvement.

ii. e. *Mycoplasma pneumoniae.*

Mycoplasma pneumoniae is often felt to be the causative organism. Although it is quite conceivable that influenza-type viruses may also be involved, outbreaks of bullous myringitis have historically been identified in patients with atypical pneumonia from *Mycoplasma* involvement. It is also possible that the bullous eruptions may represent a nonspecific reaction to an underlying otitis media.

81 e. tubal granuloma.

A tubal granuloma is the most likely diagnosis in the above scenario, which appears to develop in approximately 1–2% of patients with a ventilation tube (grommet). Histologically, it is postulated that implantation of keratin debris in the ventilation tube provokes a classic foreign-body-type granulomatous reaction. Treatment usually requires tube removal. In some circumstances, combination topical antibiotic–steroid drops may be used to settle the inflammatory response. Care is required, however, if potential ototoxic medication is used in the presence of a TM defect (in this case secondary to the ventilation tube). Oral antibiotic therapy generally plays no significant part in the treatment of a foreign body reaction.

82 a. granular myringitis.

Granular myringitis represents a localized chronic inflammation of the TM characterized by the presence of granulation tissue. As the middle ear is not involved, hearing should be relatively normal, and a type A curve would be expected on tympanometry. Treatment requires identification of the aetiological agent by bacterial or fungal culture. Appropriate antimicrobials are often combined with frequent microdebridement of the ear. In recalcitrant cases, surgical debridement under anaesthetic may be required.

83 i. a. true.

An acute diffuse external otitis ('swimmer's ear') is typically caused by *Pseudomonas aeruginosa.* As a general rule, exposure to moisture and local trauma (e.g. scratches in the ear canal) are the most frequent predisposing factors. Treatment generally involves local debridement, the occasional insertion of a wick to stent the ear canal open, and the appropriate selection of topical antibiotic–steroid drops or a solution that will acidify the ear canal (*Pseudomonas* thrives in a basic pH environment).

ii. b. fungal otitis externa.

The development of a secondary fungal otitis externa (otomycosis) is not unusual, and may follow treatment with topical antibiotic–steroid drops. The two most common organisms cultured are *Aspergillus* and *Candida* species.

iii. d. *Aspergillus niger.*

This otoscopic slide demonstrates classic *Aspergillus niger* otomycosis. The white, cotton-like threads represent fungal hyphae, whereas the black or greyish dots represent conidiophores. Treatment requires meticulous debridement and the instillation of appropriate antimycotic agents.

84 e. carcinoma of the ear canal.

The otoscopic picture is that of squamous cell carcinoma involving the external auditory canal (EAC). Extremely uncommon, the incidence of malignancy involving the EAC and mastoid is generally quoted at 0.01% of all reported neoplasms. Risk factors for carcinoma of the EAC generally include a history of chronic inflammation (e.g. chronic external otitis), exposure to radioactive substances (e.g. radon), chromate burns (e.g. from matchsticks used to clean the ear canal) etc.

The vast majority of patients with EAC malignancy present with a history of puritis, otorrhea, trismus and/or intractable pain. The pain is often described as deep, boring and unrelenting, the sinister implication being bony or dural involvement. Unfortunately, in many instances it is only when a change in the aural discharge or intractable pain occurs that the clinician is alerted to the seriousness of the disease process. Development of a facial palsy is related to tumour involvement in the mastoid. Most malignancies of the EAC in adults are squamous-cell carcinomas.

Although prognosis is generally poor, combination treatment with primary surgical excision and post-operative radiotherapy is generally advocated. Five-year survival rate for primary EAC carcinoma in aggregate series is approximately 28%.

85 i. a. eustachian tube.
    b. endolymphatic sac.
    c. sinus tympani.
    d. facial recess.
    e. basal turn of the cochlea.
  ii. b. false.
    The sinus tympani is a potential space in the posterior mesotympanum that lies medial to the facial nerve and runs from the oval window to the inferior aspect of the round window niche.
  iii. b. false.
    In canal wall-up procedures, access to the middle ear via the mastoid is provided through the facial recess. As the sinus tympani is medial to the facial nerve, any attempt to approach this structure through the mastoid would result in injury to the facial nerve or inner ear.
  iv. a. true.
    Residual or recurrent cholesteatoma is often left behind in the sinus tympani, which is a region inaccessible to the surgeon. This is one of the major causes for failure of CAT procedures.

86 a. eustachian tube.
    b. malleus.
    c. mastoid antrum.
    d. facial recess.
    e. stapes.
    f. facial nerve.
    g. modiolus.
    h. saccule.
    i. external auditory canal.

j. vestibule.

k. internal auditory canal.

87 i. e. all of the above.

By definition, a whitish lesion on the oral mucosa is termed a leucoplakia. A history of previous trauma or irritation of the oral mucosa could occur from smoking, or from local dental pathology. HIV-seropositive patients and those taking antibiotics or steroids have a high incidence of oral candidiasis that has been well documented.

ii. e. oral hairy leucoplakia.

The exclusion of candidiasis and the biopsy results are highly suggestive that these lesions represent oral hairy leucoplakia. First described by Greenspan, *et al.* in 1984, it has been clearly demonstrated that this lesion is unique to HIV-seropositive individuals. Moreover, the appearance of oral hairy leucoplakia is a good indicator that the patient will soon progress to full-blown clinical AIDS. The biopsy results essentially exclude the other listed possibilities.

iii. a. true.

Oral hairy leucoplakia occurs in 5–25% of patients with AIDS. In one prospective study of homosexual males and bisexual males with oral hairy leucoplakia but without AIDS, approximately 50% developed clinical AIDS by 18 months. By 31 months, almost 80% had subsequently developed clinical AIDS. Regrettably, the presence of oral hairy leucoplakia is a poor prognostic sign in the HIV infection.

88 i. Until proven otherwise, Kaposi's sarcoma (KS) must be considered the most likely diagnosis. KS is second only to Pneumocystis carinii pneumonia as the most frequent manifestation of AIDS.

Although KS lesions may appear on any oral mucosal surface, for some unknown reason almost 95% are found on the hard palate. Initially, KS lesions are blue and slightly erythematous compared to the surrounding mucosa. With continued growth, the lesions become elevated and often bleed from ulceration. The lesions are typically painless even when ulceration has occurred.

ii. c. 0.4%.

Compared to hepatitis B transmission from an inadvertent needle stick injury (risk estimated at 6–30%), it is estimated that seroconversion to an HIV-seropositive status occurs in 0.4% (4 in every 1,000) of injuries. The greatest risk has been associated with hollow-bore needles which deliver contaminated blood into the body. Injuries caused by a scalpel blade and suture needles are less likely to cause seroconversion. Universal precautions should always be observed. Prophylactic treatment with AZT has been recommended in cases of inadvertent occupational exposure but its efficacy remains unknown.

89 i. d. *Streptococcus pneumoniae.*

c. *Haemophilus influenzae.*

a. *Moraxella catarrhalis.*

This child is most assuredly experiencing an acute attack of otitis media (OM). By definition, OM represents an infection/inflammation of the mucoperiosteal lining of the middle ear and it is typically bacterial. *Streptococcus pneumoniae*, *Haemophilus influenzae* and *Moraxella catarrhalis* species are commonly identifiable. Although *E. coli* and *Pseudomonas aeruginosa* are possible, they are more frequently seen in neonates or children with an underlying immunodeficiency.

  ii. b. the development of a mastoiditis.
     c. presence of beta lactamase-producing organisms.
     d. viral involvement.

Failure to improve, despite compliant antibiotic therapy, may indicate that a complication such as mastoiditis has occurred, or that the underlying infection may be viral. More attention is now being focused on the increasing prevalence of beta lactamase-producing organisms (primarily *Haemophilis influenzae* and *Moraxella catarrhalis* species) that de-activate conventional aminopenicillins used in the treatment of acute OM. Antibiotic change is indicated if this possibility is suspected. Finally, in some instances, surgical drainage via myringotomy may be necessary.

  iii. b. false.

Beta lactamase-producing organisms are much more commonly identified in children than in adults.

90 i. The circular red lesion in the centre of the tympanic membrane suggests it is in contact with a vascular middle-ear lesion. The most likely diagnosis is a glomus tympanicum tumour (non-chromaffin–staining paraganglioma), either arising from the promontory or from the jugular bulb.

  ii. Routine audiological and preoperative investigations will not make this vital distinction. Plain radiographs may show enlargement of the jugular foramen, but asymmetry is a common normal finding. CT scanning demonstrates the bony erosion of the margins of the foramen and loss of the bony partition with the hypotympanum seen in glomus jugulare. The far more innocent glomus tympanicum can grow to interfere with ossicular function or compromise mastoid ventilation, but is not associated with cranial neuropathies. MRI and angiography may be useful supplements.

  iii. A tympanotomy has been performed. The posterior half of the tympanic membrane has been reflected anteriorly (to the left) to reveal the malleus handle and the long process of the incus. Crossing superficial to these is the chorda tympani. To the right (in the posterior middle ear) is the stapedius tendon above and the round window niche below. The vascular glomus tympanicum is seen arising from the promontory. It arose from chemoreceptor cells associated with the tympanic plexus.

  iv. Blanching of a glomus tumour on positive pressure pneumatic otoscopy is better known as Brown's sign. As the pressure is relieved, capillary refilling causes the tumour to assume its red colour once again.

91 i. a. physical therapy manoeuvres.
     b. vestibular sedatives.

Vestibular sedatives may provide a certain amount of symptomatic relief but, on their own, will not prevent attacks of BPPV from occurring following a provocative head movement. Most patients learn to avoid those positional movements that are associated with the onset of their spells. Physical therapy manoeuvres have recently been advocated in the hope that cupuloliths or free-flowing debris in the posterior semicircular canal may be displaced into more silent areas of the inner ear.

Diuretic therapy, low-salt diets and vasodilator therapy have no role to play in BPPV.

ii. a. singular neurectomy.

  b. non-ampullary posterior semicircular canal occlusion.

  d. vestibular neurectomy.

Although a labyrinthectomy would prove curative, it would result in a complete hearing loss in the operated ear. Endolymphatic sac decompression surgery (although controversial) is only indicated for the treatment of Menière's syndrome.

92 e. Menière's syndrome.

The histopathological finding of idiopathic endolymphatic hydrops in a patient with fluctuant hearing loss, episodic attacks of vertigo (lasting minutes to hours) and tinnitus is classic for Menière's syndrome.

It is felt that the earliest changes in Menière's syndrome occur in the scala media of the cochlea, where there is a ballooning or displacement of Reissner's membrane due to increased endolymphatic pressure. Whether this condition results from over-production of endolymph or an inability to absorb endolymph within the endo-lymphatic sac remains controversial. Progressive endolymphatic hypertension is said to cause membrane ruptures or breaks in Reissner's membrane or the walls of the saccule and utricle. According to the sodium–potassium intoxication theory, admixture of endolymph and perilymph alters the electrochemical properties and ultimately affects neural activity within the inner ear. This theory has been used to explain the hearing loss and vestibular dysfunction that occurs in patients with Menière's syndrome.

93 i. c. Vincent van Gogh.

Van Gogh's dramatic and turbulent life continues to interest and inspire those who have seen his paintings. Although ultimately he died by his own hand, there has been much speculation and many theories proposed for his often idiosyncratic nature.

ii. e. Menière's syndrome.

Recently there has been speculation that van Gogh suffered from Menière's syndrome. Some authorities have said that this condition would explain the attacks of tinnitus and dizziness that he experienced, and his erratic behaviour. Inca-pacitating attacks of Menière's syndrome may have explained why he chose to cut off part of his left ear.

94 i. d. Menière's syndrome

Non-positional, dependent, spontaneous reversals of nystagmus are commonly identified during an acute attack of Menière's syndrome. In the electronystag-mograph (ENG) tracing an irritative-type nystagmus was initially identified which spontaneously reversed at approximately 20 seconds to a deafferentiative-type nystagmus. With continued ENG recording another reversal, often termed recovery nystagmus, may have been identified. Membrane ruptures from progressive endolymphatic hydrops in support of the sodium–potassium intoxication theory, and a 'central vestibular adaptor', have been postulated to account for the nystagmus reversals in Menière's syndrome.

ii. a. right.

By definition, the so-called irritative-type nystagmus is said to be directed towards the involved side, whereas the deafferentiative-type nystagmus beats towards the uninvolved side. In most patients with Menière's syndrome, the irritative phase is short-lived, and often missed clinically. In the preceding example, the irritative phase demonstrated right-beating nystagmus that reversed shortly towards a deafferentative-type left-beating nystagmus. This would imply that the patient had a diagnosis of right Menière's syndrome. In fact, this was the clinical diagnosis which was confirmed audiometrically.

95 b. an Arnold–Chiari malformation.

The findings of occipital headache, ataxia, downbeat nystagmus in the primary position and poor pursuit in the presence of a bilateral caloric reduction require that a central lesion, specifically at the level of the cervical medullary junction, needs to be excluded. In this regard, MRI is the imaging investigation of choice. In this case, MRI confirms cerebellar tonsil herniation through the foramen magnum, which is pathognomonic for an Arnold–Chiari malformation. Note is also made of a small syrinx in the upper-cervical spinal cord.

In this hind-brain malformation it is postulated that downbeat nystagmus, a bilateral caloric reduction, poor pursuit and the subjective complaints of oscillopsia (visual blurring with head movement) are the result of vestibular cerebellar compression. Occipital headaches are not unusual in the Arnold–Chiari malformation, and are thought to arise when there is transient obstruction of the fourth ventricle that typically occurs with straining or with manoeuvres that transiently raise intracranial pressure.

Although the other possibilities listed may give rise to a number of the symptoms and signs identified in the preceding case description, the imaging features strongly point to only one diagnosis.

96 i. b. basal-cell carcinoma.

The findings in this patient are secondary to a large erosive basal-cell carcinoma. The presence of a facial palsy implies significant mastoid involvement, although the inner ear is probably not affected (based on the finding of a conductive hearing loss). As basal-cell carcinomas are relatively asymptomatic, they often go unnoticed or may be ignored for a considerable length of time. It would be extremely rare for a basal-cell carcinoma to metastasize.

Although ulceration may occur with all the other listed possibilities, it would be rare for this to occur without other signs or symptoms being present. In this regard, mycosis fungoides is typically associated with the development of lymphoma, whereas pyoderma gangrenosum is often seen in association with various systemic diseases, such as ulcerative colitis, rheumatoid arthritis or myelogenous leukaemia. A squamous-cell carcinoma is possible, but does not typically present with that degree of significant ulceration. A keratoacanthoma demonstrates a central area of necrosis, but this in itself should not be extensive.

ii. e. temporal bone resection with a composite myocutaneous flap repair.

The extensive nature of this ulcer requires a formal temporal bone resection which will leave a significant composite defect in the lateral skull base. As a result, a composite myocutaneous flap repair is required that can either be performed with an axial myocutaneous (e.g. latissimus dorsi, trapezius) or microvascular-free (e.g. rectus abdominous) flap. There is no role for a modified radical or a radical mastoidectomy in the treatment of this extensive and erosive condition. Advances in reconstruction have made rotational scalp and local myogenous flap repairs obsolete in the reconstruction of a significant lateral skull base defect.

97   c. facial nerve schwannoma.

History of recurrent facial paralysis in association with a conductive hearing loss requires that a facial nerve schwannoma involving the horizontal (tympanic) segment of the facial nerve must be present. Imaging studies utilizing both CT and MRI technology provide valuable information concerning bone and soft-tissue involvement respectively in the middle ear.

In general, glomus jugulare tumours arise from the jugular bulb in the region of the inferior hypotympanum, and result in a 'rising sun' appearance of the tympanic membrane (TM). Although obliterative otosclerosis may cause a reddish hue to the TM in the posterior superior quadrant (Schwartz's sign), it should not cause facial paralysis. Acoustic neuromas are associated with a progressive sensorineural hearing loss and tinnitus. They typically begin in the internal auditory canal, and usually expand into the cerebellar pontine angle. Rarely do they erode into the middle ear. Finally, an aberrant internal carotid artery would be most unusual in this anatomical location, although a persistent, enlarged, stapedial artery is theoretically possible.

98   Cochlear implantation is, of course, a possibility. The audiogram on first inspection suggests that stapedectomy could not help, and that there is no residual hearing. She has given no response to bone conduction testing, and the limited AC threshold may well be vibrotactile. There is, it seems, no cochlear function.

This pessimistic view may be correct. However, the audiogram is taken from a genuine case who underwent a trial of stapedectomy with a very rewarding outcome.

Indeed, she has given no response to bone conduction testing, but this investigation has its limits. BC stimuli are limited by the outputs of the equipment. In this case, 60 dB is the maximum output at each frequency, and she has failed to respond. What if her true thresholds are 70 dB for bone conduction? A stapedectomy that eliminates conductive loss may raise her air conduction levels to that level, and makes a hearing aid a very viable proposition. A conductive deafness requires far more amplification than the 'half gain' applied to a similar degree of sensorineural loss.

This 'hidden bone conduction' did, after all, indicate a greater cochlear reserve than audiometry could hope to quantify.

99   i. The left nasal ala shows the characteristic cutaneous lesions of hereditary haemorrhagic telangiectasia, or Rendu–Osler–Weber disease. Similar lesions will arise in the mucosa of the alimentary tract and upper respiratory tract. AV malformations are commonly found in the lungs and central nervous system (CNS). Haemorrhage from any of these sites is a major problem, and repeated epistaxes the rule.

    ii. Complications of the disease include GI haemorrhage, haemoptysis and cerebro-vascular bleeds. Pulmonary shunting may compromise the cardiovascular system. Acute blood loss leads to hypovolaemia, chronic blood loss to anaemia. Repeated transfusions caused increasing difficulties with sensitization and risk of blood–bone infections such as hepatitis B and HIV. Excessive iron administration may cause haemochromatosis.

100 The initial impression is of a profound, mixed, hearing loss with a marked conductive component at low frequencies. An optimist might feel that surgery to correct, for example, a congenital ossicular disorder could improve hearing to a level where a hearing aid could be used.

    The wary specialist will appreciate that the audiogram does not ring true. There is an impossibly wide air–bone gap at low frequencies and none at high frequencies. The bone conduction symbols on the right do not represent thresholds, but are the limits of machine testing, reached without a response.

    This patient has not, in fact, produced a single audiometric response. All thresholds are felt, rather than heard, and most patients with no cochlear function could produce this audiogram.

    Surgery is not totally excluded. A pre-lingually deafened young adult with no auditory memory is not an ideal candidate for cochlear implantation.

101 i. There is overinflation of the left lung with mediastinal displacement. This is due to partial obstruction of the left main bronchus by a foreign body. The ball–valve effect causes outflow obstruction, a consequent wheeze and 'air-trapping'.

    ii. Alveolar distension will be worsened by any ventilatory measures. A sudden deterioration in clinical condition could be the result of:
- mediastinal emphysema;
- tension pneumothorax;
- displacement of the foreign body distally with complete obstruction.

    Mediastinal emphysema will ultimately be associated with subcutaneous crepitus but will not respond to routine measures for treatment of pneumothorax. A tension pneumothorax is of course easily mistaken for an overinflated lung.

    Positive pressure ventilation is to be avoided, therefore. Such measures as ventilating the opposite lung or apnoeic oxygen diffusion down the bronchoscope allow a speedy removal of the foreign body.

102 The suspicion here was a preseptal cellulitis secondary to maxillary sinusitis. After intensive antibiotic treatment, he was taken to the operating theatre the next day for sinus washout. Prior palpation of the swelling produced a gush of pus from the lacrimal punctum and immediate resolution of the swelling!

    This patient had acute dacrocystitis, and the overlying soft-tissue swelling has produced the hazy appearance on the sinus radiograph. In retrospect, the marked submandibular lymphadenopathy and the involvement of the lower rather than the upper lid suggests the diagnosis.

103 i. In an Oriental patient presenting with significant cervical lymphadenopathy, a nasopharyngeal primary carcinoma, with nodal metastasis, is immediately suggested.

ii. Nasopharyngeal carcinoma may be quite extensive before producing localizing nasal symptoms. A painless lymphadenopathy is a common presenting feature.

Obstruction of the eustachian tube may lead to middle ear effusion which is always a worrying feature in an adult. A conductive hearing loss results.

Invasion of the skull base and cavernous sinus can produce cranial neuropathies. Damage to the upper cranial nerves causes diplopia, visual loss and hemifacial pain or anaesthesia. Lower cranial nerve damage causes dysphagia and dysarthria. Direct tumour extension can cause proptosis or palatal distortion. Distant metastases may supervene.

In this patient the expected diagnosis did not emerge. Neck exploration was rewarded with a gush of pus from what proved to be a cold abscess!

104 e. cholesterol granuloma.

When enhancing lesions are demonstrated on both T1 and T2 weighted MRI sequences in the temporal bone it is almost pathognomonic for a cholesterol granuloma. Although a dehiscent jugular bulb is the only other condition listed clinically that would give a blued appearance to the tympanic membrane, it would not enhance and would not be typically associated with a flow void signal.

Cholesterol granulomas are thought to arise when a bleed occurs under the mucoperiosteum in the middle ear. Cholesterol from degenerating erythrocytes gives rise to a chronic foreign body granulomatous type reaction. The high density of hydrogen ions in cholesterol is though in part to be the reason why a bright signal enhancement occurs in both T1 and T2 weighted images. As there is no actual tumour present it would be unlikely for this lesion to enhance following gadolinium injection.

105 i. • Very rare.
• Slow growing.
• Difficult to biopsy—this could be misleading.
• Symptoms include dyspnoea, hoarseness, dysphagia or a sensation of a lump in the throat.
• Histological grading is difficult. Malignancy is confirmed by the biological behaviour.
• Radio resistant.
• Treatment is surgery.
ii. Total laryngectomy, because of the large size of the tumour and the extent to which it had involved the cricoid. A near-total cricoidectomy or wide local excision would not have been possible in this patient.

106 i. • Congenital abnormalities, e.g. lymphangioma, haemangioma.
• Neck abscess, e.g. parapharyngeal abscess, Bezold's.
• Hamartoma.
• Choristoma.
• Teratoma.
• Neoplasm, e.g. rhabdomyosarcoma.
• Lymphadenopathy, e.g. scrofula (TB), diphtheria.
ii. • Mechanical upper airway obstruction superior to the site of tracheostomy.

ANSWERS

- Access to the lower respiratory tract for bronchial cleansing.
- Respiratory failure, e.g. coma.

The indication in this case was for a mechanical obstruction caused by a lymphangioma (cystic hygroma).

107 i. Syphilitic osteitis of the skull base on the left. Soft-tissue density material in both middle-ear clefts.
    ii. • Congenital syphilis, e.g. sabre tibia.
      • Acquired tertiary syphilis, e.g. periostitis of the calvarium in syphilis.

108 In the case of normal CSF:
    a. Penicillin G, 24 million units intravenously per day × 10–14 days.
    b. Benzyl penicillin 2.4 million units once a week × 2 after completion of above.
    c. Probenecid 500 mg b.d. during the time that penicillin is given.
In the case of positive CSF:
    a. As above, but limited to 10 days.
    b. As above.
    c. As above.
    d. Amoxicillin 3.5 gm orally daily with probenecid for 60 days after the completion of a–c.
    e. Prednisone 80 mg alternate mornings × 1 month, and then reducing regime over two weeks.

109 i. Leprosy is a disease occurring in tropical and subtropical regions. It is an infective condition dcaused by *Mycobacterium leprae*, also known as Hansen's bacillus.
    ii. Ridley and Jopling described five clinical types based on the host's cellular immune response:
      1. Tuberculoid (TT) — Paucibacillary and delayed hypersensitivity
      2. Borderline tuberculoid (BT)
      3. Borderline (BB) — Multibacillary and anergy
      4. Borderline lepromatous (BL)
      5. Lepromatous

110 i. It is an autosomal-recessive disorder of unknown aetiology.
    ii. • Hyaline-like deposits in the dermis and submucosa.
      • Fragility of the terminal blood vessels from birth.
      • Hoarseness.
      • Macroglossia.
      • Stomatitis and gingivitis.
      • Alopecia and loss of eyelashes.
      • Intracranial deposition with secondary calcification (hippocampal region).
    iii. • Plastic surgery for unsightly skin lesions.
      • Genetic and psychological counselling.

111 i. • Facial paralysis.
      • Oedema of the lips and cheeks.
      • Cheilitis.

- Furrowed tongue.
ii. As for idiopathic facial paralysis, i.e.:
  - Prednisolone 60 mg per day for 4 days, reducing by 5 mg each day until a dosage of 5 mg per day is reached. Continue with this dosage for 10 days. Total duration of the treatment will be 25 days;
  - Facial nerve decompression if indicated on electro–neuronography;
  - Protection of the involved eye against drying and corneal ulceration.
  The aetiology is unknown, hence management is symptomatic.

112 i. c. squamous-cell carcinoma.

The finding of a fungating mass on the lower lip associated with palpable lymphadenopathy in the submental and submandibular regions bilaterally indicates a squamous-cell carcinoma until proven otherwise. A biopsy is definitely required for histopathological confirmation.

ii. c. polycystic kidney disease.

The development of squamous-cell carcinoma and lymphoma in the upper aerodigestive tract has been well documented in post-transplantation patients who receive immunosuppressive therapy. As a general rule, the longer a treatment course with immunosuppressive agents the more likely a secondary malignancy will occur. Other associated risk factors include the subject's occupation as a farmer (from a presumed exposure to the harmful effects of ultraviolet radiation) and his pipe smoking/oral tobacco use (thermal irritation and the carcinogenic effects of tobacco). Polycystic disease on its own would not ordinarily be a causative factor.

113 Vision should be tested. It is possible that the patient may have an impairment of which they are unaware. Should they become aware of it after the operation, they may erroneously blame the surgeon for causing the problem.

114 i. d. *Pseudomonas aeruginosa.*

Otoscopy reveals classic evidence of a diffuse external otitis that is better known as 'swimmer's ear' (despite the negative history of swimming). *Pseudomonas aeruginosa* is usually identified as the causative organism. This gram-negative bacterium appears to thrive in a basic pH environment. Microdebridement and local treatment with topical antibiotic–steroid drop combinations or preparations that acidify the EAC are commonly used. When the EAC is diffusely swollen, a wick is usually inserted which acts as a vehicle carrier so that the drops may reach the deep recesses of the canal. Oral antibiotics are generally efficacious in the treatment of this gram-negative infection, although ciprofloxacin has shown some promise.

ii. b. Diabetes mellitus.

Recurrent attacks of both bacterial and fungal external otitis are not unusual in diabetes. Appropriate investigations are therefore required to exclude the presence of this disorder. A number of immunological defects have been identified in diabetics. The most important of these are:

- poor leucocyte migration at inflammatory sites leading to relative leucopenia and overall impairment of cellular defence mechanisms;
- diminished activity of neutrophils, macrophages and monocytes in the presence of ketoacidosis and hyperglycaemia.

- marked reduction in lymphocyte reactivity to standard nitrogens (substances that promote lymphocytic activity), especially in the presence of hyperglycaemia. On a cellular level, such defects complement our knowledge of the ischaemic and the micro–angiopathic changes that occur in diabetics and offer an explanation of why these patients are predisposed to bacterial and fungal infections.

115 Lepromatous leprosy. The features are:
- Diffuse skin involvement with almost no areas of unaffected skin.
- Diffuse nerve involvement of the extremities.
- Loss of eyebrows.
- Marked ENT symptoms.
- Multiple bacilli on skin smears.

116 The demonstration slide shows an osseointegrated, bone-anchored hearing aid and artificial pinna in place. The illustration on page **85** shows the side of the head with the prostheses removed.

117 i. a. bone-marrow biopsy.
     d. radionuclide skeletal survey.
     The presence of proteinuria, significant monoclonal serum proteins, hyper-calcaemia and a clinical history of numerous pathologic fractures suggest that a diagnosis of multiple myeloma (MM) needs to be primarily excluded. A bone-marrow biopsy would confirm the presence of an increased number of abnormal, atypical or immature plasma cells. A radionuclide skeletal survey would document localized involvement in other skeletal areas and assist as a guide for the bone biopsy site. Plasma cell reaction secondary to connective tissue disorders, liver disease metastatic carcinoma and the entity of benign monoclonal gammopathy would be rare, considering the clinical scenario presented.
     ii. d. multiple myeloma involving the cricoid.
     Via a laryngofissure approach, this subglottic mass was removed, thereby confirming the presence of an intracricoid plasmacytoma. Considering the systemic involvement of this disease process, a diagnosis of multiple myeloma (MM) appears most likely.
     Although a diagnosis of an extramedullary plasmocytoma (EMP) could be made if this was a solitary lesion, it is important to realize that both EMP and MM are probably part of a continuous disease spectrum. In this regard, nearly 30–70% of patients with a localized EMP are identified as having evidence of MM on further investigation.
     Treatment for MM mainly requires appropriate chemotherapy. In this case description, the patient underwent surgical excision, which was followed by post-operative radiotherapy (200Gy × 10 fractionations over two weeks). To date, no laryngeal recurrence has been identified.
     Although a functioning parathyroid adenoma may produce hypercalcemia and skeletal lesions, it is not associated with plasma cell infiltration or abnormal monoclonal proteinuria (Bence–Jones). Primary biliary cirrhosis and Wegener's granulomatosis present primarily with other symptoms.

118 i. e. A carotid angiogram with balloon occlusion/xenon washout test.

Given the circumstances, the finding of multiple acute-onset cranial nerve palsies (VII, VIII and X) requires that an infective process involving the skull base needs to be excluded. The development of a fulminant skull base osteomyelitis has been well documented in diabetics, patients with haematological malignancy or those with previous irradiation to the skull base in whom external otitis or mastoiditis has proven difficult to treat. A carotid angiogram with balloon occlusion/xenon washout test is not indicated in this condition unless a temporal bone resection was contemplated. Initial investigations would include biopsy of granulation tissue and culture of the discharge. This is necessary to exclude the remote possibility of malignancy or to identify the causative organism for a skull base infection. Blood glucose measurements and urinalysis will help to determine whether a patient's diabetes is under control (which is mandatory for the treatment of any infection). Finally, a high-resolution CT scan will demonstrate whether intracranial sup-puration is present in the form of an abscess or whether there has been erosion into the otic capsule.

ii. a. gallium–67 citrate radionuclide scan.

Radionuclide scans mirror the metabolic changes that occur in bone and therefore are important in determining whether an infective process has occurred. Technetium^{99m} uptake occurs in bone as a result of any nonspecific osteolytic/osteoblastic reaction and, in essence, reflects increased blood flow to the involved area. This technique, however, has limited specificity for osteomyelitis, and any condition causing osteogenic activity (neoplasms, arthritic disorders or skeletal trauma from surgery) will have similar uptake patterns. Moreover, it is not unusual for a scan to remain positive for several years, even after the clinical resolution of the underlying condition.

Complementary scanning with gallium–67 citrate is recommended, as this radionuclide is actively taken up and highly concentrated in the lactoferrin complexes of white blood cells. Uptake of this radionuclide in the suspect region would indicate active infection, thus confirming a skull-base osteomyelitis. Indium-labelled white blood cells have also been used (see illustration on page **86**) to provide confirmation of infection.

119 i. Because the differential diagnosis includes the following:
- Chronic specific infection, e.g. TB, syphilis.
- Neoplasms, e.g. lymphoma, leukaemia, squamous-cell carcinoma, adeno-carcinoma.

ii.
- Low-grade.
- Intermediate-grade.
- High-grade.

iii.
- External radiation.
- Chemotherapy.

120 i.

Leukaemia type		ENT symptoms
1. Acute lymphatic	1.1	Leukaemic infiltrate in the oral cavity, e.g. gums
	1.2	Ulceration and bleeding
	1.3	Pharyngitis
2. Chronic lymphatic	2.1	Cervical lymphadenopathy
	2.2	Tonsillar enlargement
3. Chronic myeloid	3.1	Epistaxis ++
	3.2	Bleeding from other mucosal surfaces
	(3.3	Splenomegaly)

 ii. • High index of suspicion and clinical findings.
   • Haematological assessment.
   • Biopsy.

121 i. Black hairy tongue.
   This is seen in the following situations:
   • Prolonged use of systemic antibiotics.
   • Antiseptic mouthwashes, e.g. chlorhexidine.
   • Oral mycoses.
   • Colourants in refreshments and foods.
   • Tobacco smoking.
 ii. • Red tongue, e.g. scarlet fever, allergy.
   • White-coated, e.g. thrush, diphtheria, non-specific stomatitis.

122 i. • Pressure necrosis due to an ill-fitting dental plate.
   • Allergic reaction to the denture material.
   • Ulceration of an underlying torus palatinus.
 ii. • Male.
   • 6th decade.
   • A long history of progressively enlarging swelling in the parotid gland. 80% of these tumours are in the parotid.
   • A firm, nodular tumour.
 iii. Wide local excision and careful follow-up.

123 i. • Unknown.
 ii. • Localised areas of the tongue lose their filiform papillae and appear to be a brighter red than the surrounding areas of normal tongue surface.
   • The denuded areas change periodically in site and size. Adjacent areas may coalesce.
   • Painless.

iii. No treatment is required.Care must be taken, however, not to confuse this condition with other pathologies of similar presentation, such as the mucous patches or 'snail-track' ulcers seen in secondary syphilis.

124 i. Ranula.
  ii. Retention cyst due to obstruction of a sublingual gland duct. This is usually spontaneous, but may be the result of trauma or surgery to the floor of the mouth. Re-routing of the submandibular duct (Whartons's duct) in cases of excessive drooling may develop a ranula as a post-operative complication.
 iii. • Marsupialization.
      • Excision including the sublingual salivary gland from which it is arising.

125 i. • Pyrexia.
      • Rigours.
      • Myalgia and arthralgia.
      • Tachycardia.
      • Malaise.
      • Headache.
      • Abdominal pain, often with vomiting in children.
  ii. • Inflamed and enlarged tonsils.
      • Purulent exudate or whitish membrane on the tonsils.
      • Coated tongue, foetor oris, referred earache.
      • Dysphagia.
      • Trismus.
 iii. • Acute follicular tonsillitis.
      • Acute parenchymatous tonsillitis.
 iv. • Scarlet fever.
      • Diphtheria.
      • Infectious mononucleosis.
      • Agranulocytosis.
      • Leukaemia.
      • Lymphoma.
      • Secondary syphilis.

126 i. d. Ludwig's angina.
      The picture that accompanies the case description is compatible with an expanding haematoma involving the floor of the mouth and tongue. If this was an infection, it would be compatible with a condition called Ludwig's angina. This represents a rapidly spreading floor-of-mouth cellulitis that may ultimately cause airway obstruction. The progressive stridor and dysphagia are indeed worrisome and, when these occur regardless of cause, an alternative airway is often required (via nasotracheal tube intubation or a formal tracheotomy). Although supraglottitis (a more extensive form of epiglottitis) causes both progressive stridor and dysphagia, it is typically associated only with laryngeal involvement. A quinsy (peritonsillar abscess) and a parapharyngeal abscess typically involve the oropharynx and generally do not involve the floor of the mouth. Vincent's angina is typically associated with ulcers involving the oral cavity. This should not lead to a rapidly spreading floor-of-mouth cellulitis.

ANSWERS

ii. c. Coagulation screen.

When this patient was assessed clinically he was found to have widespread bruising involving other parts of the body (see page **86**). A coagulation screen revealed him to have a prothrombin time (PT) greater that 5 times the expected value (normal therapeutic range during anticoagulation being 1.5–2.5 times normal). Although his airway was of great concern, he was managed by slowly reversing his anticoagulation status towards the therapeutic range.

127 a. mucocele.

The bright signal identified in this unenhanced MRI is compatible with a large ethmoid mucocele. This arose in a post-traumatic fashion following a nasal ethmoid fracture. The bright homogeneous high signal intensity is pathognomonic for this condition. Different signal intensities would be identified if this in fact represented a post-traumatic meningoencephalocele. A caroticocavernous fistula would have presented with a large flow void (dark area on MRI). An olfactory neuroma should not present in this fashion. Although a cholesterol granuloma has similar characteristics this is more often seen in the temporal bone rather than the paranasal sinuses.

For treatment, functional sinus endoscopy techniques were used to drain this mucocele internally.

128 i. e. juvenile nasopharyngeal angiofibroma.

The selected external carotid angiogram reveals an extremely vascular lesion arising in the nasopharynx that is clinically compatible with a juvenile nasopharyngeal angiofibroma.

Nasopharyngeal angiofibromas are rare, benign lesions that occur almost exclusively in males during adolescence. The most common presenting symptoms include severe recurrent epistaxis and nasal obstruction. Serous otitis occurs as the result of eustachian tube obstruction. Continued growth in the nasopharynx may lead to recurrent sinusitis, bone erosion, anosmia and progressive sinus involvement. The major blood supply to this vascular tumour is generally derived from branches of the internal maxillary and ascending pharyngeal arteries.

ii. b. false.

There is general consensus that the biopsy of a juvenile nasopharyngeal angiofibroma is unnecessary as it frequently leads to severe bleeding. Unfortunately, because of their vascular nature, their local aggressive character and their limited tendency to undergo spontaneous regression, active treatment is required for most nasopharyngeal angiofibromas. Surgical removal is generally advocated in those smaller tumours not demonstrating significant intracranial extension. Pre-operative embolization is an efficacious technique for the reduction of operative blood loss. In larger tumours (especially those with intracranial extension), radiotherapy has been successful in reported long term control of tumour growth in patients receiving between 2,500–3,000cGy. The role of hormonal therapy remains controversial.

129 i. b. primary acquired cholesteatoma.

These features are compatible with classic primary acquired cholesteatoma. Although misnamed, cholesteatoma refers to the presence of keratinizing squamous

128

epithelium in the middle ear cleft that has a propensity for secondary infection and bony erosion. Complications arise because of its proximity to the inner ear, facial nerve and brain. For this reason, surgery is usually recommended, primarily to provide for a safe and dry ear, and secondarily to improve hearing.

Primary acquired cholesteatoma is conventionally thought to arise from attic retraction pockets involving Shrapnell's membrane (pars flaccida) that result from chronic eustachian tube dysfunction. Failure of epithelial migration from the attic pocket leads to the formation of a gradual expanding sac of skin that grows along paths of least resistance.

Congenital cholesteatoma typically presents as a white mass behind an intact tympanic membrane in the anterior superior quadrant. Cholesterol granuloma, rhabdomyosarcoma and glomus tympanicum tumours are different in colour and are noted behind an intact tympanic membrane initially.

ii. c. *Pseudomonas aeruginosa.*

The pungent smell that accompanies cholesteatoma is usually the result of *Pseudomonas aeruginosa*. Keratin debris acts as a wonderful culture media for this organism which synergistically promotes further cholesteatoma growth.

iii. e. lateral semicircular canal.

Primary acquired cholesteatoma typically spreads from the attic into the aditus ad antrum and mastoid air cells proper. The lateral semicircular canal is closest to the cholesteatoma sac and is most at risk from fistula formation in the region of the aditus ad antrum and mastoid antrum. If suspected clinically, a high resolution CT scan of the temporal bone may provide radiologic evidence. Care should be taken at surgery if a fistula is suspected in order to prevent the inner ear from an injury that may ultimately result in an acute cochleovestibular loss.

130   b. an implantation cholesteatoma.

This well recognized complication of tympanoplasty surgery occurs when viable squamous cells are inadvertently implanted at surgery behind a newly constructed TM. Implantation cholesteatoma can also occur following a temporal bone fracture or result from a blast injury causing a traumatic TM perforation. Silent at first, progressive growth eventually causes this epithelial cyst to interfere with the function of the TM and ossicular chain. Unless a secondary infection intervenes, the process is usually painless. Diagnosis can be confirmed at myringotomy. Revision tympanoplasty is generally indicated. In extensive cases, an open mastoidectomy (modified or radical) or a combined approach tympanoplasty (CAT) may be required. Under the following circumstances it would be extremely unusual for a chorda tympani neuroma or a reactive exostosis to occur. Tympanosclerosis does not usually cause a bulging TM and cholesterol granulomas are typically blue in colour.

131 i. d. benign positional paroxysmal vertigo (BPPV).

The finding of basophilic staining debris on the ampullated end of the posterior semicircular canal is termed cupulolithiasis, and is thought to represent the pathophysiologic correlate of BPPV. BPPV represents the most common inner ear disorder identified clinically and exhibits bilaterality in approximately 15% of patients. It is also not unusual to see BPPV accompany other disorders of inner ear dysfunction (e.g. Menière's syndrome, vestibular neuronitis, recurrent vestibulo-pathy).

ii. d. positional-induced vertigo, lasting seconds.

Attacks of BPPV typically last for seconds, (10–30) and may occur many times a day following a provocative head movement (e.g. looking up, bending over, rolling over in bed). BPPV most often occurs on an idiopathic basis, but its presence following trauma (head injury, skull fracture, middle-ear surgery) is well recognized. Periods of remission and exacerbation are not uncommon.

132 b. acoustic neuroma.

In the histopathological slide, there is the finding of a small intracanalicular acoustic neuroma. In general, the incidence of an acoustic neuroma, clinically, is estimated at approximately 1:15,000 patients. On histopathological grounds, however, they may be more common, and various temporal bone series have reported their incidental finding between 0.5 and 1%. It is not surprising that a high-resolution CT scan did not identify this intracanalicular tumour. The resolution on CT is generally estimated to be at approximately 5 mm with regard to an extracanalicular extension of this tumour. Magnetic resonance imaging with gadolinium enhancement would be a more appropriate test if there was concern that an intracanalicular tumour was present. As a general rule, an unexplained asymmetric sensorineural hearing loss should be considered to be due to an acoustic neuroma until proven otherwise.

133 i. e. homonymous hemianopia.

The schwannoma identified on the MRI has both extensive intracranial and extracranial spread. The signs and symptoms of tumour growth in the CP angle are well-documented and, in the extreme, will involve cranial nerves V–XII. A left homonymous hemianopia therefore would be an extremely unusual event in the presence of a large CP angle tumour. When visual symptoms occur, however, in patients with large CP angle tumours, this is generally the result of hydrocephalus and secondary papilloedema, which causes a global decrease in visual acuity.

ii. a. the jugular foramen.

c. hypoglossal foramen.

The extracranial involvement of this tumour strongly suggests that it arose from either the hypoglossal foramen (hypoglossal nerve) or the nerves of the jugular foramen (glossopharyngeal, vagus or accessory nerves). Although acoustic neuromas, trigeminal neuromas and facial nerve neuromas, in that order, are the most common schwannomas to arise in the CP angle, they typically do not demonstrate extracranial extension into the skull base.

In this patient, the tumour was ultimately identified to be a hypoglossal schwannoma. It was completely removed in a one-stage lateral skull-base approach that utilized techniques involved in both translabyrinthine and infratemporal fossa surgical approaches. It is generally felt that the tumour recurred because its extracranial portion had not been excised during the initial resection eight years prior.

134 This patient suffers from spastic dysphonia, a type of dystonia. An intralaryngeal injection of 5 units of Dysport® (Botulinum toxin type A) is being administered to each vocalis muscle under EMG control, using an injecting-needle electrode. This usually produces an improvement in voice for about 9 weeks. Side-effects include intralaryngeal haematoma and dysphagia.

135 i. This patient has an anterior deviation of the nasal septum with a spur to the right. The convexity compromises the airway, which can cause epistaxis, and may be a factor in occlusion of the osteomeatal complex in sinusitis. This may be the result of trauma or a developmental problem.

ii. Submucosal resection gives reliable results even in inexperienced hands, but does risk:
- an external nasal deformity if excessive cartilage is removed anteriorly, e.g. a saddle deformity or columellar retraction;
- interference with growth of the nasal skeleton if performed before maturity;
- septal perforation if mucosal tears are in apposition.

A conservative approach is the septoplasty, which aims to re-site rather than resect cartilage. It is preferred in anterior deformities and in children, but is technically more demanding.

136 i. This patient has an oro-antral fistula. This is more common in the pre-molar and molar dentition area where tooth roots are closely related to the floor of the antrum. Symptoms are those of maxillary sinusitis with the foul smell (cacosmia) due to anaerobic sepsis. Liquids and food ascend into the antrum, and the sinus empyema drains down through the fistula.

ii. This alveolar fistula is the result of dental trauma. Surgical trauma, and especially failure of a Caldwell–Luc sublabial antrotomy to heal, may present a similar picture. Erosive disease of bone includes malignancy, syphilis, TB and granulomatous lesions.

iii. If immediately recognised, a fistula may be prevented by rotation of a local gingival flap and antibiotic prophylaxis. Once established, the epithelial tract must be removed. The ascending sinusitis will require an antrotomy. A local flap repair can be attempted.

137 d. esthesioneuroblastoma.

The finding of a fleshy, pinkish-grey mass that is associated with a predominance of neurocytes in rosette formations is characteristic of an esthesioneuroblastoma.

An esthesioneuroblastoma is a neurogenic tumour of the olfactory region. It is relatively rare, but is associated histologically with the presence of neurocytes and neuroblasts in rosette or pseudo-rosette formations. It is estimated that approximately 20% of these tumours will metastasize. There is no histological correlation with the clinical course and the cytological appearance of these tumours. Intracranial extension is not unusual. This patient ultimately underwent an anterior craniofacial resection requiring the expertise of both neurosurgeons and otolaryngologists. To date, there has been no evidence of recurrence.

The other possibilities listed are not associated with rosette formations, although they all may produce nonspecific signs that arise from tumour obstruction.

138 i. a. yes.

As a general rule, approximately 95% of patients will have resolution of a serous effusion behind an intact tympanic membrane within three months unless a secondary infection occurs. In order to improve this patient's hearing, it would have been reasonable to suggest a myringotomy and tube placement.

ii. b. posterior superior.

Although difficult to prove, it is conceivable that a myringotomy performed in the posterior-superior quadrant may have dislocated the ossicular chain and inadvertently dislodged the stapes from the oval window. It is for this reason that the posterior-superior quadrant should be avoided when a myringotomy is performed. Other complications could include injury to the chorda tympani nerve, and possibly even the facial nerve if it were in an aberrant location. It is less likely that the round window could have been inadvertently lacerated at the time of surgery.

139 i. The patient has multiple juvenile papillomatosis, here seen affecting both vocal cords.

ii. Damage to the anterior commissure (the single most common site for papillomas) has left both vocal cords denuded of epithelium, which has led to web formation. This blunting effect compromises the airway, and the voice is hoarse. Endoscopic division generally adds to the trauma and worsens matters.

If the papillomatosis resolves, a laryngo-fissure technique can be used to divide the web and allow insertion of a keel stent. This separates the cords until they become re-epithelialized, when it can then be withdrawn.

140 i. Mucormycosis (rhinocerebral phycomycosis—see illustration on page **87**).

ii. The organism has a predilection for blood vessels, which it invades, causing obstruction, thrombosis and infarction. It characteristically has non-septate–branching hyphae.

iii. • Very active control of the underlying diabetes mellitus.
  • Early and aggressive local debridement.
  • Systemic antifungal medication, e.g. Amphotericin B.

iv. Sagittal sinus thrombophlebitis causing infarction.

The cranial CT scan demonstrates a bilateral frontal lobe infarction from sagittal sinus thrombophlebitis. The darkened areas represent regions of necrosis and would also account for an obtunded state. Meningitis would not specifically localize itself to one area of the brain. There is no evidence to suggest an actual brain abscess.

141 i. c. post-cricoid carcinoma.

Until proven otherwise, the operating diagnosis must be a post-cricoid carcinoma (usually squamous-cell carcinoma). Taking into consideration the progressive weight loss, hoarseness and maternal history of carcinoma, a panendoscopy with biopsy is required.

ii. a. Plummer–Vinson syndrome.

Sideropenic (iron deficiency) dysphagia is often seen in association with the presence of oesophageal webs, angular cheilitis, atrophic glossitis and koilonychia (spooning of the finger nails). When this occurs the diagnosis is pathognomonic for Plummer–Vinson (Paterson–Kelly) syndrome.

Almost exclusively a disease of females, this poorly understood hereditary disorder is associated with an increased risk of pharyngeal and oesophageal carcinoma in predisposed individuals. When an idiopathic upper oesophageal web is identified in a patient complaining of dysphagia, it is important constantly to monitor the patient. Although the mechanism for carcinogenesis is poorly understood, it does not appear to be related to the typical history of smoking and alcohol intake noted otherwise with carcinoma of the upper aerodigestive tract. Treatment requires a combination of radiotherapy and surgery in the form of a pharyngolaryngectomy with appropriate reconstruction.

As a general rule, Zollinger–Ellison syndrome, Sjögren's syndrome, Rosenthal–Melkersson syndrome and avitaminosis C are not associated with epithelial malignancy in the upper aerodigestive tract or oesophageal web formation.

142 i. Dysplasia implies a fault in the normal maturation of epithelial cells as they progress from the basement membrane to the surface. The degree of cellular atypia is an indicator of severity. If the dysplasia affects the full depth of the epithelium but the basement membrane is intact, this is termed carcinoma in situ. The pathology report implies residual changes at the anterior commissive after surgery, possibly showing frank invasion.

ii. The natural history is uncertain. If causative factors such as smoking are eliminated, the condition may be reversible. Some will progress to invasive squamous-cell carcinoma, and monitoring is essential.

Careful outpatient examination with fibreoptic endoscopy is vital. Suspicious areas must be removed and studied, although, in this case, care must be taken to avoid damage to the anterior commissure. The CO_2 laser is useful in atraumatically treating areas of field change, but it leaves little for the pathologist to study. Persisting carcinoma in situ confirmed at repeated microlaryngoscopy is seen by some as an indication for radiotherapy. This, of course, rules out non-surgical treatment should invasive carcinoma develop subsequently.

143 a. T4 N0 M0.
b. T4, because the tumour has grown outside the larynx through the thyroid cartilage. Had it not done so it would have been a T3 primary lesion. The site of origin, i.e. whether it was originally glottic or subglottic, is unknown. It is a transglottic carcinoma.

144 i. He has left enophthalmos and a slight depression of the left visual axis.
ii. He proves to have a blow-out fracture. This is a consequence of blunt, non-penetrating injury to the globe causing a fracture of the orbital wall, herniation of the orbital contents (fat or muscle) but with an intact orbital rim. Fracture through the lamina papyracae or floor of the orbit (as here) can entrap recti muscles causing diplopia on vertical or lateral gaze.
iii. A full ophthalmologic examination, to include:
- tests of visual acuity;
- pupillary function;
- ocular mobility;
- fundoscopy (and anterior chamber examination acutely for hyphaema);

- forced duction test;
- plain radiographs and coronal CT scan.

145i. a. longitudinal temporal bone fracture with an incus dislocation.

Otoscopy reveals classic evidence of a step deformity involving the posterior superior bony external auditory canal. This is pathognomonic for a longitudinal skull fracture, and would account for the bleeding that was identified in her right ear following the accident. Otoscopy also reveals evidence of an incus dislocation relative to its position in the normal middle ear. Of interest, this patient clinically had relatively good hearing in her right ear, and audiometry demonstrated that only a mild conductive hearing loss was present. It is probably reasonable to assume that a spontaneous incus transposition occurred as a result of this accident.

ii. d. post-traumatic benign positional paroxysmal vertigo.

The findings in the Dix–Hallpike manoeuvre are classic for left benign positional paroxysmal vertigo (BPPV). This is an extremely common sequela following head injury. As a result, debris released by the trauma is thought to gravitate onto the ampullated end of the posterior semicircular canal (cupulolithiasis), or to arise within the canal proper, leading to a free-floating plug (canalith). There are no atypical features to suggest a central nervous system localization for the paroxysmal attacks of vertigo. Although a perilymphatic fistula may arise from a post-traumatic event, the positional attacks of vertigo and absence of hearing fluctuation make this possibility unlikely. Ménière's syndrome is not generally thought to arise from a post-traumatic head injury.

iii. b. unlikely.

The persistence of her attacks for two years makes it extremely unlikely that she will experience a degree of spontaneous remission. As a general rule, patients are more likely to undergo surgical treatment for this condition when it arises in post-traumatic fashion. Physical therapy manoeuvres (the so-called liberating or particle repositioning procedures) are less likely to be successful in this scenario.

146i. • Herpes zoster.
- Herpes simplex.
- Recurrent aphthous ulcers.
- Behçet's syndrome.

ii. Herpes zoster is unilateral and follows the distribution of a specific cranial nerve, e.g. V.

iii. Immunodepression, such as occurs in AIDS, promotes the development of herpes lesions. The presence of a herpes infection may be the first indication of AIDS.

iv. • Acyclovir.
- Oral hygiene, antiseptic mouth washes.
- Analgesics.
- I.V. fluid if the pain makes swallowing difficult.

147 c. magnetic resonance imaging with gadolinium enhancement (MRI–g);
d. high-resolution–enhanced CT scan.

Evoked-response audiometry measures electrical potentials in the auditory system that are elicited by sound stimuli (e.g. clicks, tone pips and tone bursts). The potentials resulting from this stimulation are picked up by electrodes, amplified and delivered to an averaging computer.

Three different electrical responses have been identified in terms of their measured potentials, latencies and site of anatomic production. These are the electrocochleogram (0–2 milliseconds), the auditory brain-stem response (0–10 milliseconds) and cortical-evoked responses (greater than 50 milliseconds).

ABR in a normal ear typically reveals a series of stable waveforms with good morphology over the first 10 milliseconds of stimulation. Abnormalities in terms of poor waveform morphology and delays in both absolute (wave 5) and interwave (1–5) latencies are highly indicative of a retrocochlear disorder such as an acoustic neuroma.

Sophisticated imaging studies that demonstrate an enlargement of the internal auditory canal (IAC) or a soft tissue mass in the IAC/cerebellar pontine angle are usually required to exclude or confirm the presence of an acoustic neuroma. In this regard, both high-resolution–enhanced CT and MRI–g scans are complementary, and are required especially if surgical removal is indicated. Digital subtraction angiography (DSA), carotid doppler studies and radionuclide scans have no role in the conventional investigations of an acoustic neuroma.

148 b. noise-induced deafness.

The finding of a sensorineural hearing loss associated with a characteristic notched appearance between 3,000 and 6,000 Hz is almost pathognomonic for noise-induced hearing loss. A bi-product of civilization, both occupational and non-occupational noise may ultimately result in deafness that is largely preventable with appropriate hearing protection.

Exposure to loud noise initially results in a temporary threshold shift (TTS) that is largely reversible and thought to reflect metabolic injury at the level of the cochlea. Continued exposure, however, eventually results in a permanent threshold shift (PTS) that is irreversible. Noise levels that are specifically greater than 90 dB during an average working day of eight hours may eventually cause hearing loss in susceptible individuals.

Specific examples include:
- rocket launchpad   180 dB
- jet plane   140 dB
- gunshot blast   140 dB
- automobile horn   120 dB
- pneumatic drill   100 dB
- subway   90 dB
- average factory   85 dB
- noisy restaurant   80 dB
- conversational speech   65 dB
- average home   50 dB
- soft whisper   30 dB

In order to minimize occupational hearing loss, legislation has been passed that limits employees from working in loud noise unless appropriate hearing protection is worn. Although regulations vary from country to country, as a general rule, with each 3dB increment in sound intensity levels above 90dB, the acceptable length of exposure to noise is halved. This is demonstrated in the table **below**.

Sound in dB	Duration (hours per workaday acceptable)
90	8
92	8
95	4
97	3
100	2
102	1½
105	1
110	½
115	¼ or less
115+	no exposure without hearing protection

Source: Section 144 of Ontario Regulation 714\82
Occupational Health and Safety Act. (OHSA)

149 The figure shows papilloedema. In the presence of chronic otorrhoea, a brain abscess must be excluded.

150 i. • Destruction of the anterior nasal septum.
     • Three perforations of the palate. The largest one involves the hard palate, whereas the two smaller ones are situated in the soft palate.
  ii. Syphilis, a highly contagious disease, caused by an infection with *Treponema pallidum*, a spirochaete.
  iii. a. Congenital syphilis due to intra-uterine infection.
      b. Acquired syphilis.
     • Stage 1 - primary chancre, painless ulceration and lymphadenopathy.
     • Stage 2 - mucous patches, condylomata, papillo-squamous rash and lymphadenopathy.
     • Stage 3 - Gumma, 15 years after the primary infection. It has preference for the hard palate.
         - Neurosyphilis with meningitis, otosyphilis.
         - Osteitis.

151 c. metastatic malignant melanoma.
The dense brown discolouration involving the facial nerve in the geniculate ganglion and its labyrinthine segment is pathognomonic for metastatic malignant melanoma. Histologically, malignant melanoma is characterized by an increased

number of atypical and bizarre melanocytes that have a propensity for metastatic spread. The brown discolouration arises from particles of melanin in the cytoplasm of the malignant cells. In all probability, it would be extremely rare for a remote cutaneous squamous-cell carcinoma to metastasize to the temporal bone. Lesions in Kaposi's sarcoma are typically bluish in nature, tending to affect mucosal and cutaneous surfaces. Although brownish discolourations of the skin (café-au-lait spots) are identified with NF1, this condition is not typically associated with the development of facial or acoustic nerve schwannomas. Lesions in NF2 may involve both the facial and cochleovestibular nerves, but they are non-pigmented and are histologically compatible with benign schwannomas.

INDEX